JUICING
For Authentic Balance
MISTY ANGELIQUE

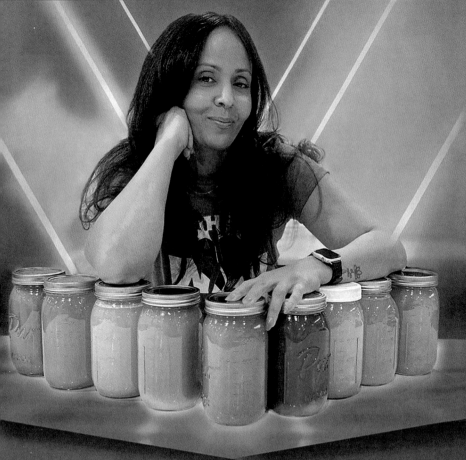

THE EXACT PLAN THAT I USED TO BRING
AUTHENTIC BALANCE
BACK INTO MY LIFE!

To My Wonderful AB Community:

I warmly invite you to immerse yourself in all that *The AB Way* has to offer during this season of your life. Similar to what my book designer told me when she sent the first draft one evening, "It's after work hours, so don't feel pressured to review this in your off-time. *Authentic Beauties* need *Authentic Breaks* too!"

I want to extend the same sentiment to you.

Oh, and *Authentic Beauty*, by the way, extends beyond physical appearance and applies to both men and women. It includes qualities such as authenticity, integrity, emotional intelligence, confidence, kindness, intellectual curiosity. resilience, and strength. Men with these qualities exhibit a form of beauty that goes beyond surface-level attractiveness and resonates on a deeper level. *Authentic Beauty* should be seen as subjective, recognizing that true attractiveness stems from inner qualities rather than external appearance.

With that, no matter who's reading this, as you journey through this book, stay on your *Authentic Boulevard* and establish *Authentic Boundaries* to embrace and benefit from your *Authentic Breaks* fully. My hope is that this new way of living will ignite your *Authentic Boldness* that will lead you to *Authentic Blessings* as we become lifelong *Authentic Besties*.

From the heart.

Contents

Foreword

Hello all. I know you may be wondering who I am. I go by Nikki Marie, just so you know, but this tale has less to do with me and more about why you landed here.

We all want to be our greatest selves…
We all want to live the highest quality of life possible… figuring out how to make that happen seems to be a struggle that we all can relate to.

I've been in contact with Misty Angelique since 2012. When I had my first glimpse of her, I admired her confidence and how intellectual she was. She just always flowed, you know,

…like the waves in the ocean.

…like the birds singing in the trees.

…I always felt calm with her.

If I had known back then what I know now, I would have made sure I never lost contact with her. Misty had some health issues, and she stepped away from social media for a bit for what she now calls her wilderness experience. I'll let her tell you all about that.

What I'm here to tell you is this: From the moment she came back, I knew I had witnessed a miracle. I know that saying "miracle" sounds dramatic but listen: I wasn't awakened at the time, so for me to even notice the shift within her was a big deal. I could have been like everyone else and responded haphazardly like, "Oh, Misty's back, cool," and just continued on with my everyday life.

Instead, I made it my business to see what she was up to. In doing that, not only was I awakened, but the whole direction of my life changed. The blurred vision of my life became crystal clear, and that, my beautiful readers, is what you call alignment. Never question it. Never doubt it. Just run in the direction where you feel most alive.

It's no secret, really. I just couldn't hear or see anything because my mind and body were clogged. Misty and her Juicing For Authentic Balance System helped me to undo all of that.

For the first time in my life, I felt like my body was functioning the way it was designed to. Because you may not know much about this juicing program, it may not seem like a big deal to you, right? But for me, it's everything!

What does juicing really do for you, one may ask?

Well, let me tell you. Imagine needing glasses for years, and then finally, you get a pair. The moment you can see again, it's a beautiful thing, and a whole new world is before you.

Imagine walking through the fog when suddenly it clears up and the sun comes out. You'd probably say, "What a beautiful day! And I have a beautiful life ahead!"

Imagine having headaches from hell, and then suddenly, they become less frequent and stop.

Imagine not knowing what to do with your life, and then boom, you now have direction.

It's a beautiful feeling that I'm sure we all long for.

Juicing helped me to connect all the dots.
Juicing restored my confidence.
Juicing softened me up from being numb to all situations.

Juicing made me realize everything I ever needed was in me all along. The moment I started juicing was the moment I stopped looking outside myself for all the answers. Juicing brought me back home.

This ain't for the weak and this damn sure ain't for the lazy!

I can assure you if you're willing to dig deep and do the work or become the best student you can be, unlearn and relearn everything you've been taught…

…then you, my friend, just struck gold!

Your health is the foundation of everything. including your current position and where you want to be.

I'm down 50 pounds, and I couldn't be more proud and grateful for everything that I've been taught. This was the best gift I could have ever given to myself.

Keep going and never give up! You'd be amazed at what could happen in a year if you gave it everything you've got! Stay close to those who know what they're doing. That's your golden key! I'm happy you're here, and I hope you are too!

" *Juicing restored my confidence.* "

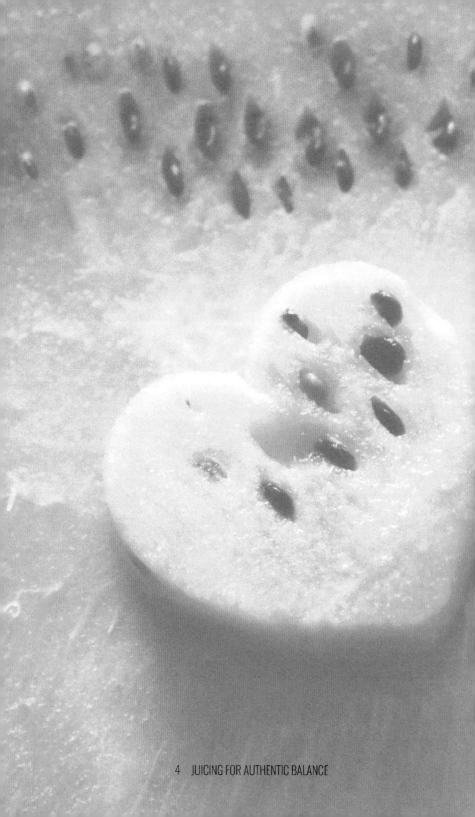

Introduction: How To Read This Book

Welcome to the AB community!

Before I explain how to navigate through this book, I'd like to introduce you to what the AB community is all about. We are a community of *Authentic Beauties* who are dedicated to *Achieving Balance* in our lives through the art of *Authentically Becoming*. Our focus is on cultivating *Authentic Bodies* through Juicing, nurturing an *Authentic Brain*, adopting *Authentic Behavior*, aiming to welcome *Authentic Bonding*, embrace our *Authentic Beauty*, and building our *Authentic Business*. So, let's get on board with *The AB way*!

This book came to fruition for three reasons. Firstly, I wanted to provide you with as much information as possible upfront, so that you will eventually work with me after being encouraged by everything you read inside. Secondly, my goal is for you to implement the knowledge given to experience results as quickly as possible so that you can apply reason number one more swiftly. Thirdly, after creating a Juicing Manual some time ago, I found that many people still had questions and desired more information about the process, which is why I decided to create a revised edition that breaks down every single detail.

As you will soon find out, throughout this book I will be extremely transparent. My team and I are here to help you, and I have structured this book strategically so that you can get a clear picture of where you want to be.

I will give you specific guidance and advice based on your current needs, and provide you with lots of material and information to ponder. I will discuss what may have put you in your current physical position, and then make a case for 'Juicing as a Lifestyle' as a way for you to put your body back into an *Authentic Balance* state.

In addition, I will discuss the myths, misconceptions, and all the ways people waste time, energy, and money on juicing that eventually led them to stop juicing altogether. I will share with you the complete Juicing For Authentic Balance System, outlining the steps and strategies that I have utilized to aid individuals in losing weight, treating health conditions naturally, or discontinuing medication. Additionally, I will highlight the items that should be immediately eliminated from your diet, the fruits and vegetables you should purchase to begin a successful juicing journey, what to expect during the juicing process, and the optimal time to implement new techniques based on your personal transformation.

Overall, this book can be summed up in three points: Juicing is a great way to get your body back in a homeostasis state; by understanding what caused your body to be in the condition that it's in now, you will first have to understand where and how it all originated; and the best method to truly implement this transitional plan within your life is to make it a daily habit.

This book is not just about juicing, but about designing a better life that brings you joy, peace, and fuels you physically, emotionally, mentally, spiritually, and even financially. I hope this book inspires and informs you on how to grow and improve your own life so that you can share this juicing evolution with others and inspire them along your journey as well.

If you find the information in this book hitting home and would like to start implementing some of the strategies immediately, you can book a call at **www.juicewithmisty.com**. Helping people like you start your juicing journey is what I do day in and day out. With that, I believe in you also. Cheers in advance to your success!

Authentically yours,

Misty Angelique

Part 1: The State of The AB Community Address

To ALL Of My *Authentic Beauties*, you know we must start this party off right by going over AB's Creed:

LOOK IN THE MIRROR. TAKE A GOOD, HARD LOOK. YOU ARE LOOKING AT A TRUE AUTHENTIC BEAUTY!

AUTHENTIC BEAUTIES KNOW THAT TRUE AND REAL BEAUTY COMES FROM WITHIN, AND IT RADIATES OUTWARD TO THOSE AROUND THEM.

AUTHENTIC BEAUTIES LIVE THEIR BEST, AUTHENTIC LIFE BECAUSE THEY KNOW GOD PROVIDED THEM WITH THE GIFTS NEEDED TO SHINE.

AUTHENTIC BEAUTIES ARE CONFIDENT AND COURAGEOUS. THEY HELP OTHERS LEAD THEIR BEST LIVES BECAUSE THEY ARE ALWAYS OUT TO HELP AND NOT HINDER.

AUTHENTIC BEAUTIES RECOGNIZE THEIR STRUGGLES BUT TAKE ACTION AND MAKE CHANGES.

AUTHENTIC BEAUTIES KNOW THAT BEAUTY IS BEYOND THE BOTTLE.

AUTHENTIC BEAUTIES KNOW THAT BEAUTY STARTS FROM THE INSIDE. IF YOU NURTURE AND LOVE THE INSIDE, THE OUTSIDE WILL REFLECT YOUR POSITIVITY.

AUTHENTIC BEAUTIES WILL TEACH OTHERS HOW TO LET THEIR AUTHENTICITY STAND OUT AND IMPACT OTHERS AROUND THEM AND AROUND THE WORLD.

AUTHENTIC BEAUTIES LOOK AT THE WORLD AROUND THEM AS FULL OF POTENTIAL AND POSSIBILITIES. THE SKY HAS NO LIMIT.

AUTHENTIC BEAUTIES RECOGNIZE WHAT NEEDS TO BE DONE AND GET IT DONE. THEY KNOW THAT IF THEY WANT TO BE SUCCESSFUL, IT REQUIRES HARD WORK AND SURROUNDING THEMSELVES WITH PEOPLE WHO CAN HELP THEM REACH THEIR GOALS.

AUTHENTIC BEAUTIES AIM TO BE THE BEST PERSON THEY CAN BE. EVERYONE HAS DIFFERENT TALENTS AND ABILITIES, BUT IT'S CRUCIAL TO PUT YOURS TO GOOD USE.

AUTHENTIC BEAUTIES RECOGNIZE THAT NAYSAYERS ARE OUT THERE, BUT THEY HAVE NO TIME FOR THE NEGATIVITY, FOR THEIR EYES ARE SET ON THE PRIZE.

AUTHENTIC BEAUTIES KNOW THEIR WORTH, VALUE, INTEGRITY, AND CHARACTER. THEY ARE CONFIDENT BECAUSE THEY KNOW EXACTLY WHAT THEY BRING TO THE TABLE.

AUTHENTIC BEAUTIES ARE NOT AFRAID TO TAKE A CHANCE BECAUSE THEY HAVE THEIR OWN STRENGTH, AS WELL AS THE STRENGTH OF OTHERS AROUND THEM, TO BACK THEM UP.

AUTHENTIC BEAUTIES KNOW BEING AUTHENTIC IS THE ONLY WAY TO BE. AFTER ALL, THERE IS ONLY ONE Y-O-U. SHOW THE WORLD WHAT YOU'VE GOT.

You Are An Authentic Beauty.
Don't Ever Forget It.

Chapter 1: Authentic Check

Now that we've addressed our *Authentic Beliefs*, let me illustrate the experience of Juicing For Authentic Balance. To begin, I must mention AB's app, which you'll have access to when we work together. But before we move forward, can I ask for a reality check? As I reflect on my health journey, I can't believe I'm writing this book and how far I've come. It's a true blessing and in addition, it includes my connection with you. I value connections deeply.

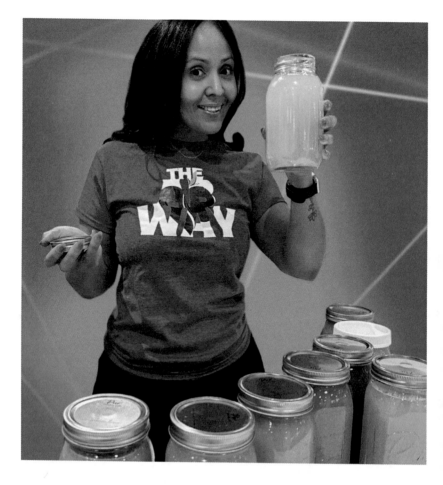

Personally, I started implementing the concepts in this book in 2019, and in 2022 I began inviting other women to join me on my healing journey while building out my health and wellness platform. Those who started with me, whom I call my Day 1's, persevered through the ups and downs of creating the system, and after applying the strategies, they saw incredible results. Many joined to lose weight, get off medication, or just to feel better overall.

After the first round of the 28-day process, the women collectively lost over 100 pounds, and a group of men joined and doubled that weight loss total. This success confirmed that the system was effective. What's even more significant is that those who accomplished their goals within the first month of the program continued to eat healthy and adhere to the plan after finishing the initial 28-day period. It's understandable, as why would anyone want to revert to their previous lifestyle after experiencing such fantastic results.

As interest grew, we had to quickly develop our backend support to accommodate demand. Throughout the initial year of implementing our program, we provided assistance to many individuals in mastering the essential concepts of juicing, as well as to those who were confronting physical obstacles.

Here are three case studies showing how juicing *The AB Way* brought *Authentic Balance* back to their bodies.

Client Case Study #1

My Dearest Nikki Marie: Let me express that Nikki is truly unique. You've already had an introduction to her in the beginning of this book and will get to know more about her and her personality when you become a member of our Facebook group. However, I would like to highlight why she has achieved such impressive results and continues to do so. Nikki is a determined individual who stays committed once she sets her mind to something, and that's precisely what she's done throughout the entire juicing process. What makes me proudest about her story is that she is experiencing everything I've outlined in this book firsthand, plus additional aspects that you will learn more about later.

In short, let's discuss authentic awakening! Nikki understands firsthand what I mean by that at this time in her life. She is now in tune with all aspects of her existence. Her story continues to astonish me, and the transformation in her spiritually guided conversations is a true indication that her life has undergone a significant shift. Of course, she has lost a significant amount of weight, but what I admire most about her situation is that the shedding of the extra weight has also resulted in the shedding of things that were holding her back and causing confusion in her life. I'm thrilled that she can now see things that were previously hidden from her, and I'm eager for her complete story to be shared. This is only the beginning!

I am fortunate to have Nikki's support in different facets of my business. It is a privilege and a source of gratitude to work with her, as she not only understands the intricacies of the juicing process but has also experienced a noteworthy personal transformation through our effective proprietary method.

Client Case Study #2

My Dearest Kim: We all understand the pressure of life's demands, especially when holding a high-level position in the corporate world. However, Kim faced an additional challenge with high blood pressure, which went undetected until she stumbled upon a home blood pressure monitoring kit. She was taken aback by the elevated readings, and after repeated tests, she visited her doctor, who confirmed the diagnosis.

Knowing the importance of kidney and adrenal health, I recommended a combination of herbs and a juicing regimen to regulate her blood pressure. Within two weeks of following the routine, her blood pressure was under control. While she wasn't keen on taking medication, she made a personal choice to prioritize juicing and lifestyle changes instead. Just to clarify, I do not recommend skipping prescribed medication. It was entirely her choice to prioritize her commitment to juicing and making a complete lifestyle change.

> " *This is only the beginning!* "

Client Case Study #3

Lauren's case was exceptionally distinctive, with her test results indicating imbalances in several areas including high blood pressure, cholesterol, triglycerides, and thyroid levels, among others. However, her six-month success story after embracing juicing is a remarkable turnaround. Following a check-up with her doctor, Lauren called me with excitement, having achieved normal ranges for certain categories, which she couldn't even remember the last time she had achieved.

What thrilled Lauren the most was the realization that her body no longer craved unhealthy foods that she was used to eating. She continues on this journey, and I encourage her to "Juice Up" even when she doesn't have an appetite for food. I explained that although appetite fluctuates during the juicing journey, it is essential to keep flushing out toxins from the system and provide the necessary nutrition. Now juicing is her go-to no matter what. Lauren sends me pictures throughout the day for accountability purposes, even when she doesn't have an appetite, continuously replenishing her body with pure goodness. She now affirms, "I always have juice or fruit on hand, no matter what."

Juicing has the potential to transform your lifestyle in numerous ways, which I will delve into shortly. The results from our AB's progressive juicing strategy speak for themselves, owing to its simplicity. While others may have struggled with juicing and maintaining consistency during cleansing efforts in the past, those committed to making it a lifestyle continue to experience tremendous benefits.

We maintain high standards for changing lives through the power of juicing, turning away around 35% of those who reach out due to our pre-qualifying process which entails commitment level requirements. We do this to ensure the ultimate success of our clients. Many people approach us with great enthusiasm, thinking they are ready for the program, but then life happens, and excuses lead to unsatisfactory outcomes.

The AB community takes change, juicing, and authenticity seriously and recognizes their powerful healing potential. We aim to help everyone experience this life-transforming process by working with those ready to implement strategies immediately, with no excuses, games, or fluff.

This book outlines the crucial factors and strategies involved in juicing for cleansing in a clear and concise manner. My simple method and the approach I follow is straightforward: by juicing, you initiate a cleansing process, which in turn leads to healing, allowing for weight loss, treatment of particular conditions, and/or reducing medication. The AB method covers these top three factors, which most people consider when adopting juicing as a lifestyle.

Incorporating a juice a day could be the simple solution you've been searching for to achieve consistent results, and this book will provide all the necessary information to unlock the answers you've been seeking. Reading every word should take less than a week (and that's stretching it). Once you delve into this crucial information and start applying, you won't want to stop. You'll continue juicing until you reach a point where you're asking yourself, "What's next? How can I continue this journey for the next year?"

By following my lead, you'll authentically awaken to some hard-core truths that will radically change your entire existence. So, if you're ready to make a commitment to this transformational journey, let's go!

Chapter 2: Who This Book Is For

The technique that you are about to discover originated during one of the most difficult times in my life. Let me elaborate...

On August 3, 2016, my life took a turn that marked the beginning of a total transformation. While I won't delve into all the intricate details between then and now, I encourage you to watch a video blog that I recorded in 2017.

However, before you do that, I must warn you. When I look back at that video, it reminds me of two things: how unwell I was and how much I have learned since then about the things that I discussed in the video. Keep in mind that I was new to my healing journey, and I was desperate to learn as much as possible in order to feel better. Despite seeking and acquiring a lot of information, as I mentioned in the video, I only experienced moderate and unsustainable success. Although I thought I was on the right track, I would often go to bed feeling miserable and wake up with a knot in my stomach, trying to identify the symptom that was troubling me in my first waking moments. I was worried about facing another day filled with constant stress and frustration, and I even experienced my first episodes of anxiety, not knowing what was happening to me.

To watch my health vlog, visit **www.myhealthstruggle.com**

It was a terrible experience. I was unable to take care of myself, or let alone work. It felt like a never-ending nightmare. Throughout that horrible ordeal, this was my first lesson: I made the mistake of overwhelming myself with too much information, buying numerous books, taking multiple supplements, and implementing countless techniques and strategies, causing my body to detoxify too quickly. As a result, I experienced die-off symptoms, making it impossible to get through each day. I was in too deep within the detoxifying process and did not know how to reverse it.

Like many others, I made the mistake of attempting to detoxify my body too fast to achieve quick results. I made too many changes at once, causing my healing process to fluctuate based on my ability to endure the stress I was placing on my body. My sleeping patterns were irregular, leading to high levels of stress.

To add to my struggles, I reached my breaking point when I discovered that I had parasites, despite doing everything I knew how to do to improve my health. I will delve into this further in part three, but the short version is this: during a visit with my colon hydrotherapist, who I went to discuss my ongoing misery with, she immediately noticed mucus coming out from my bowels as she began flushing me out and stated, "YUP, parasites!" That was it for me. It was truly a breaking point. I HAD ENOUGH and couldn't take it anymore!

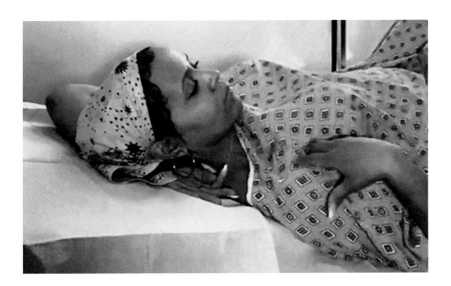

Before my physical state deteriorated beyond repair, I was fortunate to discover a Juice Certification Program. Inquisitive, I enrolled only to learn more after reading about significant health changes that others were experiencing. Once I started applying, my current state began to change slowly but surely. The simple method that I will describe in this book saved my sanity, reduced my stress levels, and allowed me to return to peak physical health. By implementing the strategies outlined in the coming pages, I achieved two significant improvements.

One, after implementing the strategies outlined in this book, my results became more reliable, measurable, and predictable within just a few days. I now have a solid understanding of what foods to eat, what to avoid, and how to juice in order to achieve specific results. Whether I want to slim down or gain a bit of weight, I have mastered different techniques that allow me to tune in to my body's needs. While my ultimate goal is to achieve total health and well-being, it's still satisfying to know exactly what to do in order to get the results I desire.

If you can't say the same about the regimens, diets, cleanses, or detox processes you've tried in the past or are currently using, it might be a sign that you need a more consistent and predictable approach to bring your body back to homeostasis. What better way to achieve this than by returning to the Garden of Eden and providing your body with all it requires by juicing fruits and vegetables? This book will teach you how to do just that.

In addition, due to the predictability of my results, I am now able to identify individuals who lack the necessary focus, motivation, and excitement to not only begin but also sustain this process, regardless of the challenges. Therefore, I make a deliberate effort to avoid any distractions from individuals who are not as dedicated to making a change as I am. I prioritize staying focused on my personal goals because I value and prioritize my own well-being, and I cannot work harder than someone who claims to desire change. Achieving remarkable results requires teamwork and commitment from both of us. I have put in too much effort to reach where I am today, and I cannot afford to regress.

The focus of this book is to teach you effective juicing strategies that deliver both predictable and scalable results, as well as help you become aware of the additional transformations that come with juicing as a lifestyle. My aim is not only to help you improve your physical health but also to help you experience the joy that comes with this journey. The unique benefits of juicing will give you an advantage over those outside our community, and you will have the knowledge to help others in the right way with the right methods that yield the desired outcomes. Ultimately, your own results will put you in a better position to help others, which is what life is all about, isn't it?

The techniques presented in this concise transitional guide are ideal for those in search of inner equilibrium. My ultimate goal is that by perusing the forthcoming pages, you will discover a route to not only achieve physical prosperity but also enhance the overall tranquility in your life. It is pointless to restore your body to optimal health if you are unable to relish life to the fullest extent in a significant manner. Therefore, my dear readers, this book is suitable for anyone seeking genuine growth and willing to undertake it in the appropriate manner.

Key Takeaways

Many people tend to rely on traditions and passing fads to achieve their desired outcomes, but this approach often results in mental and physical exhaustion and fails to produce long-term progress. Rather than following the latest trends or man-made beliefs, it is crucial to understand your *Authentic Body* and establish a lifestyle that incorporates cleansing techniques, allowing you to consistently achieve favorable outcomes even on days when you are not actively thinking about it.

The purpose of this book is to assist you in constructing a system that promotes predictable results through an enjoyable method, known as Juicing for Authentic Balance (the real JAB, if you know what I mean). This method is highly effective for individuals seeking to detoxify their bodies, shed weight, address specific health issues, or reduce their reliance on medication. I crafted this book with you in mind, and I am excited to witness the outstanding results that you will achieve from implementing these strategies.

Success Check-In Exercise

Before delving into the remainder of the book, let us first evaluate your current physical status. To accomplish this, I have created an online success check-in tool tailored exclusively for you. The tool will prompt you to rate the accuracy of a series of statements on a scale of 1 to 5, with 1 indicating "not at all accurate" and 5 indicating "highly accurate." After assessing each statement, the tool will calculate your scores and provide suggestions for your next steps.

To access the online success check-in tool, please visit **tool.juicingforauthenticbalance.com**. This tool is entirely confidential and does not require any personal information or opt-in. It is solely a self-assessment designed for your benefit.

" You will discover a route to not only achieve physical prosperity but also enhance the overall tranquility in your life! "

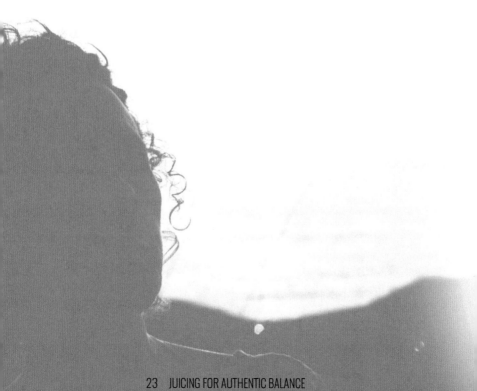

Chapter 3: Three Authentic Truths

As I mentioned earlier, my journey towards healing commenced in 2016. During this challenging period, my mother remained by my side, bearing witness to every obstacle I encountered. Despite feeling as though her words went unheard, she never ceased to encourage me. One day, amidst my frequent hospital visits, she arrived with a decorated glass bowl, a sticky notepad, and a pen. She referred to it as my "Thanks Living Jar" and instructed me to jot down things I was grateful for in every waking moment. She assured me that this was all part of my journey and that, one day, I would be able to support numerous women going through the same struggles I was experiencing at the time.

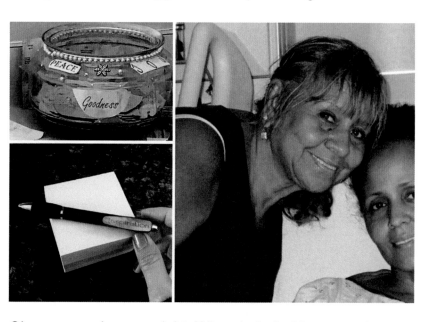

Oh my, was she ever right. When I started to recount my journey, I had no idea that numerous women would surface in different online forums, social gatherings, media outlets, and on my social media channels, revealing that they had experienced identical symptoms to mine. The sheer number of women who reached out after hearing my story convinced me to continue delving into the intricate details of my journey. After suffering from poor health for more than seven years, I've undoubtedly learned a thing or two—lessons that could only be obtained through trial, error, and repeated attempts. I'd like to share the three hard lessons I've learned in my healing journey with you for two reasons:

Firstly, so that you can learn from my mistakes and avoid repeating them.

Secondly, I want to expand further into why I am so passionately committed to juicing and why I wholeheartedly endorse it, not only for its cleansing, healing, and weight loss benefits, but also for its ability to unlock dormant potential. Trust me, just stick with me and you will soon grasp what I am conveying. Having said that, let's now explore these *Authentic Truths*:

Authentic Truth #1: Complexity Doesn't Work

Over the past few years, I've received numerous inquiries from people who wanted to try juicing after hearing about my journey and success on various platforms. Like me, they had big goals for their personal transformations, and so they dove into juicing. However, they soon encountered a problem: it didn't seem to work. Let me clarify. It wasn't that juicing itself was ineffective; rather, it was the methods and strategies they used that didn't produce the desired results. Some were also holding onto approaches from previous attempts, thinking they would work this time around. Unfortunately, that didn't pan out, and the bigger issue was that they didn't understand why.

However, the issue was not that juicing was ineffective. The problem stemmed from the fact that they were attempting to implement their own beliefs and approaches with a new method, which were not successful, or they were clinging to techniques from prior attempts, assuming they would yield the desired outcomes. Although these tactics were unsuccessful, the bigger concern was that they did not understand why.

In reality, juicing to cleanse is a science, and if the methods are not correctly applied, it can impede effective cleansing that stimulates the body to heal and/or lose weight, particularly if non-serving patterns that led to your current state are still present.

What went wrong? That's the question. Regrettably, many individuals believe that the more intricate a process is, the more effective it will be. However, the opposite is true. Complexity can make things unclear and confusing, causing us to become lost in the labyrinth of details. Consequently, it becomes more challenging to distinguish what is effective and what is not.

I can relate to this because I too made the mistake of complicating and stressing my healing process unnecessarily. As an example, consider the documented video I shared with you earlier in this book. I listed some of the things I was doing to speed up my healing, but I ended up taking in so many things that I couldn't tell what was helping me and what was making me feel worse.

The confusion led me to become discouraged and my symptoms became harder to identify. I thought this was just part of the healing process, not realizing the significance of die-off symptoms and healing crises, and why it's crucial to take things slowly. We'll go deeper into this topic later on.

After watching the video, I shared at the beginning of this book, you can probably see that I was always trying out new and different things. Books and herbal supplements were regularly arriving at my doorstep, prompting my family to inquire, "What did you order now?" Anytime I modified my meal plan, they would question, "What are you experimenting with this time?" I can't blame them for being confused because I frequently changed my approach, making my healing journey needlessly complicated and stressful.

But let's get straight to the point: healing is simple. Period. We tend to make things more complicated than they need to be for various reasons, as if simplicity doesn't exist. Remember, the more complex a system is, the less likely it is to work, and the more difficult it is to determine why.

Similar to the individuals I had spoken to who desired to juice for results but struggled, I also faced challenges in determining what was effective and what was a waste of time.

After a while, I reached a breaking point and became exhausted with the constant fluctuations and uncertainties. However, unlike the others, I refused to give up. As we move forward into the specifics of how everything eventually played out, I will provide more detailed information on the exact steps to take.

As of now, it is important to understand that my success came from being persistent and maintaining a regular routine. By simplifying my approach and implementing the methods that I will discuss in detail, I was able to achieve significant results at the start of 2021. In fact, I was able to achieve more progress within a year of following the simplified methods than I had in the five years prior.

The takeaway here is that simplicity is effective! Through my personal guidance and assistance in the Juicing For Authentic Balance program, I have consistently witnessed this principle prove true with each individual.

Later on in this book, I will explain my straightforward approach to juicing for cleansing. However, if there is one takeaway from this book, it is my hope that you develop a willingness to simplify your approach to cleansing and detoxing. By doing so, you can strengthen yourself physically and gain greater mental clarity, surpassing your current beliefs or doubts. This brings me to my next point.

Authentic Truth #2: Your Skepticisms Are NOT Welcome Here

It may sound blunt, but I need to emphasize this fact. I have heard countless excuses from individuals who express their skepticism towards clean eating, especially when it involves incorporating more fruits into their diet. If I were paid a penny for every such excuse, I would have made lots of money just by hearing these negative thoughts. It's both fascinating and disheartening to see so many people doubt the notion that pure, clean eating can be a sustainable lifestyle that promotes us thriving as humans.

In my opinion, this skepticism often prevents many people from incorporating more fruits and vegetables into their diet, despite being told about their benefits for years. While I have nothing but love for those who are skeptical, I must emphasize that what I have to offer may not be suitable for them. The plan I'll be sharing is straightforward and precise in terms of what needs to be eliminated and what needs to be added to restore balance to the body. We must acknowledge that in order to alter our present circumstances, we must stop perpetuating the negative behaviors that caused them.

The reason why we can no longer continue with our old ways are simple—just take a look at our surroundings. Toxins are present everywhere in our environment, from harmful chemicals in products and air pollution, to toxic buildings and radiation emitted by electronic devices and cell towers. Even the food we eat contains chemicals that are detrimental to our health. As such, I'm here to change this narrative for a few reasons.

Clean eating is something I advocate for, but let me be clear: it doesn't mean you have to eat "bland food" all day long. You can still enjoy your favorite treats, including baked goods, just be sure to incorporate more of the right ingredients instead of processed ones. The key is to follow the right process, which I'll be guiding you through in our time together. But it also means being aware and open-minded about what's happening in the world.

I highly recommend clean eating as much as possible, but let me clarify that it doesn't require you to eat boring or flavorless foods all day long. You can still indulge in your favorite snacks and desserts, like baked goods, as long as you choose the right ingredients instead of processed ones the majority of the time.

During our time together, I will guide you through the correct procedures that you need to follow. But be ready, because there is a lot to cover when it comes to maintaining our physical health. With that, let me take a moment to recognize and commend you for investing time in exploring your inner self during this stage of your life.

It's truly admirable and indicative of your appreciation and care for yourself.

In the same breath, our bodies want to be healthy. It's natural inclination towards health implies that most of the symptoms we experience are our body's way of carrying out its intended function. How powerful! It's essential to understand that our bodies are constantly trying to eliminate various obstacles in order to restore balance. The reality is that our bodies have been attempting to manage the toxic load we've been exposed to, and therefore, we must take steps to reduce this load. This includes being mindful of what we consume on a regular basis if we want to maintain or recover our health. Toxins not only overwhelm the body's ability to eliminate them, but they also contribute to a decline in optimal health.

What a complex situation we have here. Additionally, the healthcare system seems to focus primarily on treating symptoms rather than promoting wellness, which I believe is flawed. We've become experts at managing symptoms, but that approach is no longer beneficial for ourselves, our loved ones, or even society at large. Personally, I no longer want to be an expert in symptomology and believe that we need to shift our focus towards a more holistic approach to healthcare.

Relying solely on medication for relief, only to find that your health continues to decline, is not a sustainable way to live. I realize that you may have been disappointed in the past, and this has left you feeling skeptical about trying new products, services, or programs that promise similar outcomes.

This is understandable, as many people have been burned by false promises in the past. However, it's important to recognize that the world has become less trusting and more skeptical, but you don't have to adopt this mindset. I am here to help guide you back to fundamental principles and practices that can improve your overall health and well-being.

Despite any doubts you may have, we should appreciate the opportunity we have to embrace the juicing movement and achieve *Authentic Balance* in our bodies. Juicing can transform our lives for the better, but we must adopt it as a lifestyle rather than a temporary fix. If you've been hesitant to try juicing in the past, I believe it's important to overcome that skepticism and take another chance on yourself.

By prioritizing your own health, you'll be better equipped to serve others, even if they don't yet realize they need your help. In these challenging times, it's likely that many people are struggling and could benefit from support. It's important to remember that everyone needs help and to prioritize our own well-being so that we can be of service to others.

In practical terms, this means that you should anticipate skepticism and take steps to address it head-on. The first step is to recognize the reality of our polluted world and the challenges it presents to our health. It's important to commit to creating a plan that specifically addresses these challenges and to approach this new reality with an open mind. If you don't plan for the current climate of skepticism, your attempts to improve your health may ultimately fail. You may find yourself at a crossroads where you must confront the fact that the strategies and advice provided by medical professionals are not effective. It's a sobering truth, but one that must be acknowledged to move forward.

The truths presented in this chapter reflect the reality of what I witness on a daily basis. If you take a moment to reflect on your own life, you may recognize that some of the patterns I describe resonate with your own experiences. Despite repeating these patterns, you haven't achieved the level of health and wellness you desire. You don't have to take my word for it; simply take a look at the current state of your life and how long you've been struggling with these issues.

You may have already recognized the truth in these words. Waiting for your current approach to miraculously fix things won't help you overcome skepticism. If you're stuck in the same old habits, you won't make any progress.

Few people in the medical field avoid discussing this issue because they lack a genuine solution. In this book, not only will I show you how to overcome skepticism in today's world, but I will also guide you in discovering your authentic self along the way.

We'll talk more about that later, but for now, let's talk about the third authentic truth.

Authentic Truth #3: Be Open To Unlearning To Relearn

Let me start this one off by jumping right in. I want to dive straight into some topics that may challenge what you've been taught so far. Throughout our journey together, we'll be exploring areas such as the food pyramid that you learned about as a child, the practices and operations of the food industry, how the medical industry instructs us on treating symptoms, the natural healing and detoxification process of the body, the advantages of certain foods versus medication, and so on. These are just a few examples, but I'm sure you understand what I'm getting at.

I want to emphasize that once we connect, your life will be transformed forever. Throughout our journey, I will reveal ideas that may challenge your beliefs. I have never been one to conform to the status quo. I have always been curious and asked the question, "Why?" I strongly believe that without understanding our purpose, we cannot perform at our best since we are operating with limited knowledge. Asking "Why?" is a simple yet powerful question.

Many times, we go through situations without understanding the reason behind them, simply because we have been conditioned by propaganda. As we connect, my duty is to serve you, starting today, during this critical moment in your life. It is never my intention to offend or be controversial. That's why when people ask me questions, I always check if they prefer the unfiltered version or the diluted one.

My approach is very specific because I have found that many people claim to want the truth, but when they are confronted with it, they often cannot handle it. My goal is not to prove anyone wrong, but rather to encourage people go deeper within themselves and find the answers that have been there all along. I believe that we have the ability to prevent many of the challenges we face in life by addressing them directly, rather than waiting until we are desperate for a solution.

As we have discussed in the previous authentic truths, there are many benefits to being open to new perspectives and approaches. However, there is still one obstacle that many struggle to overcome, which we will address in the next chapter.

" ...without understanding our purpose, we cannot perform at our best... "

Chapter 4: The #1 Misconception Around Juicing

I enjoy using my juicing techniques to achieve my desired outcomes, whether they are physical, mental, or even spiritual, as they are all interconnected. While we will dive into the science of juicing in the next chapter, I want to mention here that several studies have demonstrated a connection between daily juicing and overall health, particularly with the brain.

Juicing encourages brain-body communication, which enhances your ability to attain overall fulfillment. It's no wonder that many people feel fantastic and have a lot of energy when they incorporate juicing into their daily regimen.

To me, juicing meets all of our needs. However, as I mentioned in the previous chapter, many individuals encounter one specific problem or misconception when attempting to incorporate juicing into their lives, which we will address in this chapter. Simply put, many people claim that juicing is a lot of work, and this is the root cause of their disappointment.

I can see why individuals would have this misunderstanding before becoming a devoted juicer. When I first began juicing, I looked around to see how others were incorporating juicing into their lifestyles and how coaches or business owners were teaching their methods to educate others. I was taken aback by the lack of clarity provided to those who were truly seeking solutions for various physical ailments.

Let's be clear: juicing is excellent to implement regardless of the circumstances. Elaborating on my company's mission, I am dedicated to not only juicing myself, but also teaching my techniques to others so that they can achieve the benefits of *Authentic Balance* that align with their current and desired lifestyle.

Before moving on with this topic, let me share a fun fact about how my company came to manufacture its own juicer. It's quite comical, really, because I never expected to enter the kitchen appliance industry. My background was in manufacturing beauty products, starting with hair care and moving onto skincare. But as you learned in earlier chapters, my health crisis led me to branch out into the herbal supplement market to help others avoid the mistakes I made when seeking out the right supplements to aid in healing. You'll learn more about AB's month-to-month path of herbs in chapter 8. But for now, back to the topic at hand, the inception of Authentically Branded's Juicer.

After experimenting with numerous juicers available in the market, I found one that was comparatively better than the others. Although it was not perfect, it provided a more satisfactory experience. I decided to reach out to the manufacturer and asked for a discount code to share with those who were interested in juicing and were inquiring about the juicer I was currently using.

When I asked the company for an affiliate link to share with my community, they provided me with only a 10% discount code. It was at that moment that I decided to explore manufacturing a juicer that met my particular criteria, so that my community could not only benefit from it but in conjunction offer affiliate deals to share the love with everyone.

When it came to the design details, I had specific requirements, such as compact size, quiet operation, easy assembly, usage, and cleaning, as well as the ability to produce dry pulp and plenty of juice. However, the sample machines I tried did not have enough motor power or produced pulp that was too wet. After multiple attempts, I eventually discovered the right machine, which gave rise to AB's Juicer. I would like to mention that during the writing of this book, I am in ongoing discussions with my manufacturing company about introducing a smaller, more portable juicer, as well as a larger one, as many in my market have expressed interest in these options. I am eager to see where this leads us!

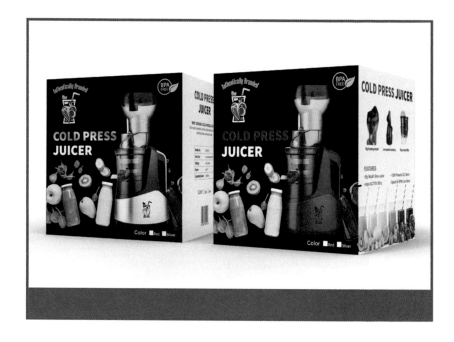

Side note: I want to express that my vision reaches beyond my personal gain from the sales of juicers. While I am a business owner and generating sales is a part of that, my true joy comes from helping others succeed. My ultimate goal is to assist individuals in achieving authentic freedom, starting with their physical health and extending it to every aspect of their lives. While it's true that I may benefit financially from my offerings, my primary focus is on empowering people to live their best lives. A juicer is a crucial component of my Juicing for Authentic Balance program, as it enables individuals to experience its full benefits. Once you've reaped these significant rewards, you'll be well-equipped to share them with others and earn a living in the process.

With the previous topic addressed, I trust that it is becoming apparent from the preceding and forthcoming chapters that my aim is to establish all-inclusive resources for my community. As previously stated, this transcends the realm of juicing, and my objective is to build a valuable foundation of sustainability for my community. Though my initial focus is on promoting health and wellness through proper juicing techniques, my ultimate aspiration is to furnish direction and assistance towards accomplishing desired lifestyle objectives. I am committed for life to making BIG things happen within the AB community!

Juicing is a significant part of my life, it has literally transformed every part of me, and I personalize the process to fit each individual's specific needs. There is no one-size-fits-all recipe, and I recommend produce based on each person's goals and health concerns. For example, my approach to juicing for someone trying to lose weight would be different from someone trying to manage diabetes with medication. I take a strategic approach and aim to address the root of the problem. Although I occasionally post beautiful juices and offer promotions, my primary focus is on providing guidance towards a specific goal.

My focus is on educating people about the body's healing abilities and how to support it through nutrition. While specific juices, herbs, and supplements can be used for targeted needs, they are not necessary at the beginning. I've learned through experience that it's important to keep things simple, especially when starting out. Unfortunately, many people have been led to believe that juicing is difficult, but I advocate for using it as a tool for cleansing and healing, which is actually quite simple. The problem lies in people's lack of knowledge, inconsistency, and failure to drink enough to see results and long-term benefits.

When I first started juicing, I immediately recognized the power of building a community around it. A community that raises awareness, encourages and informs people about the healing benefits that come with consistent juicing. As a leading juice cleansing program in the industry, I understood that if we wanted this method to make a lasting impact and change lives, we needed to reinvent the introduction to juicing by educating people about juice cleanses and the proper way to juice on a regular basis.

Today, my team and I speak to new individuals every day about the importance of having a complete juicing system in place, regardless of their lifestyle. We demonstrate how starting to incorporate juicing is easier and more beneficial than meal prepping because you obtain more nutrients from juicing fresh, living foods as opposed to cooking where most nutrients are lost due to high temperatures.

To attract engaged individuals who are excited to juice, I searched for the most active and involved members to join our community. We educate them to the point of execution and spend less than three hours per week, which includes an hour and a half for two juicing sessions typically scheduled on Sundays and Wednesdays to take care of the entire weeks' worth of juicing.

I recognize the significance of staying active and engaged when it comes to juicing, as it has transformed my life in a positive way. The individuals in our inner circle group, who are satisfied clients, follow our system without overcomplicating it. They make the most of their investment and stay consistent, preventing any long-term challenges or inconsistent behavior.

In the upcoming chapter, Part 2 of this book, I will touch on the power of juicing and its numerous benefits. I will provide an in-depth analysis of the ins and outs of juicing.

Key takeaways from this chapter are that most people have the wrong idea about juicing, their strategies are slow and unpredictable, and they spend too much time trying to achieve results without implementing the right techniques. Therefore, I have completely revamped the juicing model and introduced my method of Juicing for Authentic Balance.

My method ensures quick and predictable results, and only requires 3 hours of juicing per week, enabling people to attain new results every day. In Part 3 of this book, I will share AB's method in its entirety.

" *Juicing encourages brain-body communication, which enhances your ability to attain overall fulfillment.* "

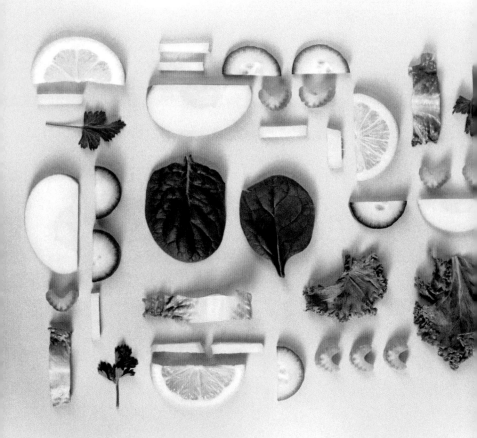

Part 2: All Things Juicing

Chapter 5: The Power Of Juicing

Have you given juicing a try? If so, great! You've likely experienced firsthand the numerous health benefits that juicing can offer. If not, get ready for an exciting journey as juicing has the potential to transform your life in many ways. However, it's essential to comprehend the fundamental principles of juicing, and this section of the book aims to help you do just that.

Juicing has become one of the fastest-growing and most popular health trends in recent times, as evidenced by the increasing number of juice bars opening up everywhere. This is a positive sign that people are becoming more conscious of the impact of their food choices on their health and overall well-being.

A recent article published in *PubMed* titled, "Overfed but Undernourished: Recognizing Nutritional Inadequacies/ Deficiencies in Patients with Overweight or Obesity" states, "Overweight and obesity are highly prevalent throughout the world and can adversely affect the nutritional status of individuals. Studies have shown that many people with obesity have an adequate intake of iron, calcium, magnesium, zinc, copper, folate and vitamins A and B12, likely as a result of poor diet quality."

Regrettably, this is just one of numerous publications over the last few decades indicating that many of us are overfed and undernourished due to our consumption of unhealthy foods. While fresh vegetables and fruits are essential for our health, providing the vitamins and enzymes our bodies require to thrive, we still fail to consume adequate amounts of these foods, leaving us feeling depleted and nutrient deficient.

Our modern diet, filled with processed sugars, flours, unhealthy fats, and cholesterol-laden foods, has weakened our bodies instead of sustaining them, leaving us vulnerable to diseases and draining our energy. In combination with a lack of exercise and exposure to environmental toxins, juicing provides a valuable weapon against the challenges of modern-day living.

Fresh vegetables and fruits are crucial to getting our health back on track, forming the foundation of our diets and enjoyed in various ways every day. Increasing our intake of fresh produce can benefit us all, and juicing offers concentrated wholesomeness that can enhance our health. A single glass of juice can contain the nutritional equivalent of several pieces of produce, providing us with essential vitamins and minerals that keep us healthy and energized.

While it's crucial to consume more fruits and vegetables, sometimes our lifestyles make it difficult to obtain the necessary amounts. Juicing solves this problem by providing a simple way to consume, enjoy and reap the benefits of fruits and vegetables several times a day. It has been shown to reduce the risk of specific cancers, heart disease, high cholesterol, and high blood pressure. Eating more than five servings of fruits and vegetables every day is recommended, and juicing makes it easy to achieve this goal.

As an illustration, drinking two cups of carrot juice, which is very doable, is equivalent in nutrition to eating eight pounds of carrots. However, it's not practical or enjoyable to consume that amount of carrots in one sitting, whereas drinking two cups of juice is easy and pleasant. Juicing can be a wonderful and convenient "fast food" option, providing a quick, highly potent, and nutritious meal.

Here's how it works: a juicer separates the liquid from the fiber and discards the latter, resulting in a highly concentrated fruit and vegetable juice. In contrast, a blender blends the whole fruits or vegetables but retains the fiber. So, what distinguishes juicing from blending, and do they both offer benefits? These are good questions.

With the current popularity of juicing, it's essential to understand the differences between juicing and blending. Juicing, as we have discussed, isolates the juice from the fiber, resulting in a concentrated amount of plant-based nutrients. Your body can quickly absorb a heavy dose of vitamins and minerals, as if you were receiving an IV infusion.

According to Juice Guru: Take a Digestion Break

"Your stomach spends six to eight hours breaking down solid foods before your cells can even begin to absorb the nutrients. Juice, on the other hand, is essentially predigested by your juicer, which extracts the nourishing liquid from the solid fibers. As a result, juice spends as little as 15 minutes in your stomach before its nutrients are available to feed your hungry cells and relatively little effort is required on the part of your digestive system to extract the nutrients. Your juicer does the hard work of breaking down the plant cells and liberating nutrients, such as minerals, carotenoids and polyphenols, that are otherwise bound to the structural components of your fruits and veggies. That leaves you with plenty of energy to spare."

When you blend a fruit or vegetable, it transforms into a liquid smoothie form, but it remains the same thing. For example, blending a carrot will give you a carrot smoothie, which is not as concentrated as juice obtained through juicing. However, blending retains the fiber that is removed during juicing. So, while juicing provides a concentrated dose of nutrients, blending offers the benefits of produce along with fiber.

The retention of fiber in blended drinks slows down absorption into the bloodstream, in contrast to juicing, which floods the system immediately. Let me explain this further.

Fiber is a crucial component in fresh foods, as it plays multiple vital roles in our health. It assists in the removal of toxic waste from our colon, prevents cholesterol from entering our bloodstream, creates a feeling of fullness after eating, aiding in weight loss, slows down sugar absorption into our bloodstream, which is particularly problematic for those with diabetes or pre-diabetes, and improves digestive functions in general.

However, juicing separates fruits, vegetables, and fiber, as the juicer pulverizes the produce into a concentrated juice and removes much of the fiber. In a sense, a juicer processes the food in the same way that processed foods have their nutrients removed, which means the juicer takes over the food processing from our digestive system.

It's undeniable that juices offer the nutrient-rich calories that our bodies need, which is why juicing is highly beneficial. It enables us to obtain the advantages of nutritious vegetables that we might not consume otherwise.

Take kale or spinach, for example. You may not relish their flavor and, as a result, avoid incorporating these essential veggies into your diet. However, when juiced together with other ingredients, you can derive significant benefits from these powerhouse foods in a much more enjoyable manner.

Harvard School of Public Health writes: "There are many types of dietary fibers that come from a range of plant foods. It's important to not hyperfocus on a particular fiber because of its specific proposed action, as each type offers some level of health benefit. Therefore, eating a wide variety of plant foods like fruits, vegetables, whole grains, legumes, nuts, and seeds to reach the fiber recommendation of 25 – 35 grams daily best ensures reaping those benefits."

Eating, juicing, and blending various fruits, vegetables, and plant foods are all beneficial for our health, and this is emphasized in the Juicing for Authentic Balance transitional plan, especially in the early stages of the cleansing process which is explained in detail in Part 3 of the book. While juice fasting, the absence of fiber allows for quicker nutrient absorption, supporting the body's cleansing and healing process by giving the digestive system a break.

It's important to note that juicing should be a part of a healthier lifestyle for maximum health and energy, and both juicing and smoothies have their uses depending on our goals. While fiber is important, the focus here is on the ability of juicing to cleanse and heal.

> " *Juicing has become one of the fastest-growing and most popular health trends in recent times...* "

Chapter 6: Detoxifying By Juice Cleansing

Do you remember that little citrus reamer that your grandmother used to make you fresh orange juice? It may surprise you, but Grandma was actually juicing! Although juicers have come a long way since then, that little gadget can still be useful at times. Our grandparents understood the importance of extracting all the nutrients from produce when possible.

Juicing is even more critical today because, let's face it, the typical Western diet is heavy in processed foods, meat, and dairy, and lacks having enough fruits and vegetables.

Here's something more disturbing found in another article published by *PubMed*, "The Western-style diet is characterized by its highly processed and refined foods and high contents of sugars, salt, and fat and protein from red meat. It has been recognized as the major contributor to metabolic disturbances and the development of obesity-related diseases including type 2 diabetes, hypertension, and cardiovascular disease. Also, the Western-style diet has been associated with an increased incidence of chronic kidney disease (CKD). A combination of dietary factors contributes to the impairment of renal vascularization, steatosis and inflammation, hypertension, and impaired renal hormonal regulation."

Oh my! Our bodies are clearly not getting the proper nutrition that's needed. Sure, when we were 12 years old, our pure energy made up for it. But as we reach our late twenties, the toll on our bodies starts to show.

Fortunately, juicing can help fill that nutritional gap. Plant-based foods contain micronutrients, the vitamins and minerals that help us feel and act our best, protect against diseases, and fight off infections. Even if we inherited great genes, we still need to protect ourselves. Think of it as inheriting gold that will rust without the proper care.

Juicing can help you achieve an *Authentic Balance* for better health. No matter your current condition, the time to start is now. Juicing is the best way to detoxify your body, reset your system, lose weight, ease gut problems, and experience extra energy you never thought possible. Trust me, I know from experience.

Let's talk about juicing and detoxing. We all know fresh produce is high in vitamins, minerals, enzymes, and phytonutrients, but the functional components of juicing and juice cleansing may not be as clear. Understanding how your body works and how juicing can benefit you is essential.

Our bodies try to detox themselves every day through urination, bowel movements, and sweating, but they need the proper fuel to do so. Our skin, liver, and kidneys are responsible for eliminating toxins, but an unhealthy lifestyle can make it difficult. Pollution, drugs, alcohol, poor diet, and the environment can create an overload of toxins that our bodies cannot eliminate naturally, leading to serious health problems.

In the past, our forefathers gathered fruits and plants while hunting for meat was less common, and no food was processed. Nowadays, we consume more processed foods, meats, fats, and dairy, turning away from what breaks down and assimilates well with our bodies (which is mostly plant-based). As a society, we are overfed and undernourished, with approximately 30% of American men and women suffering from obesity and lacking essential nutrients. We crave sugars and fats, which is not healthy. Indulging occasionally is fine, but not at the expense of flooding our bodies with proper nutrients. Junk food can become a habit, and we may not even realize it further putting our health at risk.

According to the Center for Disease Control:

"The obesity prevalence was 39.8% among adults aged 20 to 39 years, 44.3% among adults aged 40 to 59 years, and 41.5% among adults aged 60 and older. Obesity-related conditions include heart disease, stroke, type 2 diabetes and certain types of cancer. These are among the leading causes of preventable, premature death.

The estimated annual medical cost of obesity in the United States was nearly $173 billion in 2019 dollars. Medical costs for adults who had obesity were $1,861 higher than medical costs for people with healthy weight."

The statistics are concerning, but they demonstrate the significant role that juice cleanses can play in helping individuals heal, lose weight, and overcome health obstacles. Not only will they achieve their desired results, but they will also improve in other areas that they may have forgotten or learned to live with over time. I witness this transformation firsthand in the juicing world.

Juice cleansing is a powerful tool that enables the body's natural potential to heal, starting with the most critical illnesses first. It then typically heals in reverse order of when the conditions occurred, with recent conditions recovering faster than those that have persisted for a long time. This is the principle of equilibrium and homeostasis, which is true recovery. I believe it is a spiritual principle rooted in God's and Mother Nature's presence in our lives. Fasting is a powerful spiritual and natural resource that can be a miracle if you allow it to be.

While there are positive side effects of frequent or long-term juice fasting, such as increased energy, healthy hair, skin, and nails, better sleep, and a reduction in unpleasant symptoms, there are also negative side effects. As I shared earlier in my video story, I felt awful and even questioned whether life was worth living. However, I have learned that things can get worse before they get better when detoxing and cleansing. I will discuss this further later, but for now, I will say that symptoms such as night sweats, palpitations, hot and cold flashes, chills, acne, headaches, runny nose, exhaustion, body aches, and other flu-like symptoms are common. Energy levels can even fluctuate dramatically throughout the day, and it's best to go with the flow and give yourself time and space to relax when necessary.

Knowing what to expect before starting an all-juice cleanse can help you prepare mentally for any emotional or physical issues that may arise during the detoxifying process. This is what we aim to address early on in the Juicing for Authentic Balance System.

It's important to note that your experience with juice cleansing can vary from being easy and enjoyable to extremely difficult, depending on factors such as your current health condition, the types of juices you consume, your stress levels, and the duration of your cleansing journey. I often advise people not to give up on their cleanse reactions or be taken by surprise, as these unpleasant symptoms will occur regardless of whether you continue with the cleanse or remain in your current state. In fact, experiencing symptoms related to past health concerns is a common and intriguing aspect of detoxification. Therefore, the best choice is to persevere and work towards getting out of it. At least then, you'll know that the symptoms are serving a purpose.

I understand that it can be scary to go through a difficult time, having gone through it myself. That's why it's unfortunate when people prematurely break their cleanse, thinking that something is wrong or that the process isn't working. In reality, they may have given up too soon, without giving the healing process enough time to fully manifest.

I understand the struggle, but there are two realities to consider: 1). If you don't put in effort, you won't see any results. 2). If you don't understand how the cleansing process works, it can do more harm than good and leave you feeling discouraged. It's crucial to implement all the advice given, which will equip you with the knowledge to prepare for, go through, and end your cleanse properly.

By incorporating juicing into your routine, you give your body a better chance to heal. You'll soon find that you start to crave the juices, and drinking them will give you a sense of satisfaction similar to that of eating junk food. This is when you'll start to notice improvements in how you feel and look.

Chapter 7: Juice Cleansing For Specific Ailments

Differentiating between drinking juice casually and performing a juice cleanse is crucial, as a cleanse involves consuming only juices for a specific period to detoxify the body, without any solid food. However, as a Certified Juice Therapist and (W)holistic Practitioner, I must emphasize that my methods are not meant to treat, cure or diagnose any medical conditions, and it's advisable to consult a doctor before trying anything.

Before starting a juice cleanse, it's essential to prepare your body adequately, as explained in detail in The Juicing For Authentic Balance System. Gradually transitioning into the cleanse is crucial, just like how you would prepare for a marathon. You can experience significant benefits even if you start slowly.

To prepare your body for the cleanse, start by reducing your caffeine intake and incorporating more tea into your diet. Our method explains how to gracefully cut back on meat and dairy products, especially when looking to detox and cleanse. Processed foods have no health benefits and can cause several health problems, so examining labels is crucial. Beware of hidden sugars, even in foods labeled as natural.

When preparing for your cleanse, decide on your focus during the cleansing cycle, as many people embark on a juice cleanse for various reasons, such as losing weight, healing from an ailment, balancing their overall health and well-being, or getting off medication. Regardless of the reason, juicing can help achieve these goals.

Although there is more to elaborate on each area mentioned, we will touch on it more in section 3 of this book and even more within our group. Let's now move on and discuss Juicing for Gut Health.

Juicing for Gut Health

Improving gut health is one of the key benefits of a juice cleanse. As Hippocrates, the father of medicine, said over two thousand years ago, "All disease begins in the gut." Research has confirmed the significance of this statement, as an impaired gut can lead to a range of health problems, including obesity and chronic fatigue. The gut and the brain are closely connected, and when the gut is not functioning properly, it can affect our mood and overall health. Juicing is an effective way to clean up a messy gut.

A study conducted at UCLA in 2014 showed that a three-day juice cleanse can increase good bacteria while decreasing bad bacteria in the gut. People who have undergone a juice cleanse report feeling much better as it helps to eliminate toxins and restore the body to its natural state.

In addition to discussing the benefits of juicing for gut health, it's essential to provide further insight into *Candida* overgrowth. *Candida* is a type of yeast that naturally occurs in the body, and in most cases, it doesn't cause any issues. However, when *Candida* grows out of control or enters the bloodstream, it can lead to a fungal infection called *Candidiasis*. This can cause significant health problems, such as tiredness, sickness, and various other health issues.

Candida illnesses affect millions of people worldwide, and it's essential to recognize that fungal infections and yeast infections are not just a women's issue. *Candida* overgrowth can affect anyone, regardless of age or gender. By taking control of our body's internal state and improving gut health through juicing, we can prevent or manage *Candida* overgrowth and its associated health problems.

It's fascinating to observe that when people successfully control their *Candida* overgrowth, many of the symptoms and illnesses they were experiencing also disappear as they were linked to the yeast. It's incredible how interconnected everything in our bodies is, and when one thing is out of balance, it can affect the entire body in various ways. *Candida* can transform from a minor inconvenience into a harmful organism that can lead to diseases and long-term damage to the body when allowed to multiply uncontrollably.

As *Candida* multiplies and becomes systemic, it seeks out nourishment to sustain its growth. To accomplish this, it releases small roots that penetrate the gut and embed themselves into the intestinal lining of the gastrointestinal tract. "Leaky gut" is a well-known term that describes the leading cause of this condition, which results in a permeable intestinal barrier. When this barrier becomes permeable, it creates a more significant issue. The fungus and its toxic by-products can pass through the barrier and enter the bloodstream, leading to further health problems.

The book "Microbiome and Mycobiome: What in the World Are They?" is intended to be easily understood, avoiding complex medical jargon. It aims to help individuals understand what might be happening in their bodies, how to overcome this debilitating illness, and that assistance is available. However, it is essential to know some key facts about how the body works while dealing with *Candida* overgrowth. Two areas worth mentioning are the microbiome and mycobiome.

The microbiome is a collection of 100 trillion microorganisms, including bacteria, viruses, fungi, etc., that reside within our bodies. They play a crucial role in protecting us against disease-causing germs, sustaining our metabolism, and supporting our immune system. These microorganisms are essential for maintaining our health and well-being.

On the other hand, the mycobiome refers to the fungal population found in our bodies. Fungal growth can cause havoc in our bodies, and it remains an area of medicine that is still being explored. It can be frustrating to know that fungal growth contributes to or causes many diseases that impact our overall health. *Candida* and millions of other microorganisms start growing excessively when our mycobiome and microbiome are out of balance. The diagnosis of H. pylori and small intestinal bacterial overgrowth are increasingly linked with *Candida* overgrowth when these microorganisms grow out of control.

Medical Conditions Worsened With Fungal Overgrowth

As previously mentioned, excessive growth of fungi can negatively impact your entire body, leading to a worsening of existing medical conditions. *Candida* overgrowth, in particular, has been found to exacerbate a wide range of conditions, including cancers, autoimmune diseases, nervous system disorders, blood system disorders, cardiovascular issues, respiratory system disorders, digestive system disorders, skin conditions, eye/ear/mouth issues, reproductive system disorders, endocrine system disorders, urinary disorders, and viruses.

Creating The Perfect Storm For *Candida*

Candida's tendency to overgrow is not as surprising as it may seem. In fact, antibiotics play a significant role in creating the optimal conditions for *Candida* to flourish. We'll discuss this in more detail shortly.

When we consider our modern dietary habits compared to those of the past, it's important to recognize the stark differences. Our consumption of sugars, carbohydrates, dairy products, alcoholic beverages, and processed junk food is far greater than that of our ancestors who lived off the land. With our busy lifestyles, it's easier than ever to adopt unhealthy eating habits that create an ideal environment for fungi to thrive in our digestive system. Combined with the stress we experience, our blood sugar levels often increase, providing *Candida* with ample nourishment to grow and multiply. It's a perfect storm.

Antibiotics And The Role They Play

Let's return to the topic of antibiotics and their role in the overgrowth of *Candida*. While antibiotics have undoubtedly saved countless lives and are essential for treating various illnesses, it's important to acknowledge that they also contribute to the ideal environment for *Candida* to thrive. Antibiotics indiscriminately kill both good and bad bacteria in the gastrointestinal tract, which eliminates the beneficial bacteria that help keep *Candida* in check. As a result, *Candida* is free to multiply unchecked. While taking a probiotic with antibiotics can help protect the gut, it's not a complete solution.

It's worth noting that North America has relatively high rates of *Candidiasis* diagnosis, and the Journal of Infectious Diseases has identified invasive *Candidiasis* as a growing concern in US healthcare facilities. This is likely due, in part, to North America's status as the top region for antibiotic prescriptions. When yeast overgrowth occurs, it can lead to the growth of viruses, which can then turn into bacterial infections when the balance between viruses, bacteria, and fungi in the body is disrupted. This cycle continues as antibiotics are needed to treat the bacterial infection, which then kills off the good bacteria and allows yeast to grow. Other factors, such as diabetes, stress, diet, hormonal treatments, and even the chemicals in tap water, can also contribute to *Candida* overgrowth and disrupt internal balance.

Candida Of The Mouth, Throat, Esophagus

Candida overgrowth can occur in various parts of the body, including the mouth, throat, and esophagus. If you experience difficulty swallowing or pain while swallowing, it's important to speak with your doctor to rule out the possibility of esophageal *Candida*. Thrush is a common manifestation of *Candida* overgrowth in the mouth or throat, particularly in newborns.

Symptoms of *Candida* overgrowth in the mouth and throat include redness, soreness, loss of taste, the presence of white patches on the inner cheek, tongue, roof of the mouth, and throat, and pain while eating or swallowing.

Candida Of The Vagina

Both men and women can experience *Candida* overgrowth, but women are particularly familiar with vaginal yeast infections. Whether or not you've experienced one, you likely know that they are a common occurrence among women. When the pH balance of the vagina is disrupted, it creates an ideal environment for *Candida* to multiply, resulting in a vaginal yeast infection. The symptoms are difficult to ignore, and include itching of the vagina, pain or discomfort during urination or sexual intercourse, abnormal vaginal discharge, and soreness of the vagina. If you're a woman who has had a vaginal yeast infection, you know exactly what these symptoms feel like.

Invasive *Candida*

When it comes to Invasive *Candida*, the situation is much more severe compared to the overgrowths we discussed earlier. The overgrowths in the mouth, throat, esophagus, and vagina are localized to the affected area. However, in the case of Invasive *Candidiasis*, the *Candida* enters the bloodstream and can cause significant harm to the heart, brain, bones, eyes, joints, and other parts of the body. Infections of the bloodstream are the most common form of Invasive *Candida* and can be dangerous if the blood is not in a balanced state. More information on this topic will be discussed in the following chapter.

Juicing And Kidney Cleanse

Cleansing is beneficial for the body, and kidney cleanse, in particular, is essential as the kidneys are responsible for detoxifying our blood. If the kidneys do not function properly, it can lead to health problems. A kidney cleanse eliminates toxic waste that can accumulate in the blood, causing sluggishness. Before incorporating a kidney cleanse into your diet, consult with your doctor if you are on a special diet. It is advisable to start slowly to determine how to navigate through the cleansing process, especially when focusing on the kidneys.

Benefits Of A Kidney Cleanse

Cleansing is beneficial for the body, and kidney cleanse, in particular, is essential as the kidneys are responsible for detoxifying our blood. If the kidneys do not function properly, it can lead to health problems. A kidney cleanse eliminates toxic waste that can accumulate in the blood, causing sluggishness. Before incorporating a kidney cleanse into your diet, consult with your doctor if you are on a special diet. It is advisable to start slowly to determine how to navigate through the cleansing process, especially when focusing on the kidneys.

Benefits of a kidney cleanse include reduced bloating caused by toxins stored in the kidneys, decreased fatigue resulting from improper food digestion, reduced risk of kidney infections, prevention of bladder problems due to toxins or bacteria in the urinary tract, and a lower risk of developing kidney stones. Cranberry and orange juice are recommended for cleansing the kidneys as they are unfriendly to bacteria and effectively flush out kidney impurities.

> " A kidney cleanse eliminates toxic waste that can accumulate in the blood, causing sluggishness. "

Recipes For A Kidney Cleanse

Watermelon Juice

INGREDIENTS:
3 cups chopped watermelon
1 cucumber, peeled
parsley and basil leaves
the juice of 1 lemon
1 cup chopped kale
1-inch knob of ginger, peeled

DIRECTIONS: Cut the watermelon and cucumber into pieces and feed all. Process until smooth.

Cabbage Cleanse

INGREDIENTS:
½ cabbage
1 cup broccoli florets
the juice of 1 lemon
1 cucumber, peeled

DIRECTIONS: Chop the cabbage and add all ingredients to the juicer. Process until smooth.

Cranberry Juice

INGREDIENTS:
1 cup cranberries
1 cup sparkling water
2 tbsp. Matcha green tea powder
2 tbsp. honey
1 tbsp. apple cider vinegar

DIRECTIONS: Place ingredients in juicer. Process until smooth.

Watermelon Cleanse

INGREDIENTS:
2 cups cubed watermelon
1 cup blueberries
the juice of 1 lemon

DIRECTIONS:
Feed the ingredients into your juicer. Process until smooth.

Carrot Juice

INGREDIENTS:
2 carrots, peeled
2 cucumbers, peeled
½ cup of sparkling water

DIRECTIONS: Cut the vegetables in chunks and place in the juicer, along with the sparkling water. Process until smooth.

Beets and Cabbage Juice

INGREDIENTS:
2 beets
1 cucumber, peeled
½ cabbage
bunch of parsley

DIRECTIONS: Roughly chop the vegetables. Place ingredients in a juicer with enough water to help blend. Process until smooth.

Cucumber and Celery

INGREDIENTS:
3 celery stalks
1 small cucumber, peeled
¼ cup cilantro
1-inch knob of ginger, peeled

DIRECTIONS: Chop the ingredients as needed and feed into the juicer. Process until smooth.

Juicing And Anti-Aging

Aging is a natural aspect of life, and as we grow older, we begin to notice changes in our body such as sagging skin and wrinkles. While most of us desire to slow down the aging process to look and feel better, we need to understand that aging is not just about wrinkles but is a result of cellular damage and the body's inability to combat changes with enough antioxidants. Adopting a healthy lifestyle that includes optimal food consumption and a solid juicing regimen rich in antioxidants can help combat the negative effects of aging from the inside out.

In the next chapter, we will delve deeper into cleansing on a cellular level, which can be beneficial for our overall health. Consuming beet juice can help with cognitive and vascular health, while lycopene found in watermelon, tomatoes, and grapefruit has rejuvenating effects on the skin and can improve heart health by lowering LDL cholesterol and increasing "good" cholesterol levels.

As we cannot stop the aging process, being proactive in preventing the negative side effects of aging is crucial. By making small changes in our lifestyle, we can slow down the effects of aging and feel our best.

Anti-Aging Recipes

Below are some recipes that are very useful in providing anti-aging antioxidants.

Glowing Skin Juice

INGREDIENTS:
3 cups chopped watermelon
3 carrots
2 apples
1 cup blueberries
1 cup green tea

DIRECTIONS: Roughly chop the carrots and apples. Place the carrots, apples and blueberries in the juicer and process. In a glass, combine the juice and the green tea and serve over ice.

Glowing Greens Juice

INGREDIENTS:
bunch of baby spinach
1 small avocado
3 celery stalks
1 cup strawberries

DIRECTIONS: Place ingredients in a juicer and process.

Beauty Elixir

INGREDIENTS:
1 cup cranberries
1 cup blueberries
1 tbsp. sesame seeds
1 cup of black tea

DIRECTIONS: Add all ingredients except the sesame seeds to the juicer and process. Stir the seeds into the juice.

Green Sunshine Juice

INGREDIENTS:
kale leaves
collard greens
parsley
1 cucumber
1 lemon
1-inch grated ginger knob

DIRECTIONS:
Process the ingredients in a juicer.
Pour in a glass and sprinkle with cayenne pepper and turmeric.

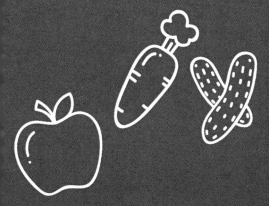

Juices For Energy

Homemade V8 Juice

INGREDIENTS:
3 tomatoes
1 onion
2 celery stalks
2 carrots
½ green bell pepper
1 garlic clove
2 cups water
lemon juice and horseradish to taste

DIRECTIONS: Roughly chop the vegetables and garlic and process all ingredients through the juicer until smooth.

Pineapple Juice Boost

INGREDIENTS:
2 cups chopped pineapple
1 orange
1-inch knob of grated ginger

DIRECTIONS: Peel the orange and place all ingredients in the juicer. Process until smooth. Serve over ice.

Kale Boost

INGREDIENTS:
bunch of kale
1 cup coconut milk or coconut water
1 chopped apple
1 tbsp. melted coconut oil
½ cup ground nuts

DIRECTIONS: Process the kale, coconut oil, chopped apple and coconut milk through the juicer. Process until smooth. If your juicer is powerful enough, add the ground nuts. If not, simply stir them into the juice.

Beet and Apple Juice

INGREDIENTS:
1 beet
1 apple
3 celery stalks
1-inch grated ginger knob

DIRECTIONS:
Feed the ingredients into your juicer. Process until smooth.

Apple Plus Juice

INGREDIENTS:
2 apples
4 carrots
1 cup spinach
1 cup broccoli florets

DIRECTIONS: Cut the apples and vegetables. Add all ingredients to juicer. Process until smooth and serve over ice.

Power Vegetable Juice

INGREDIENTS:
3 carrots
2 celery stalks
1 green pepper
1 apple

DIRECTIONS: Cut up and process the ingredients through a juicer until smooth.

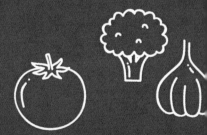

Juicing And Energy

Juicing is an incredible way to increase your energy levels, which becomes even more crucial as we age. The natural goodness of fruits and vegetables has a unique ability to revitalize and energize us.

In today's fast-paced world, most of us are trying to squeeze more than 24 hours into a single day, leading to exhaustion. As a result, many people rely on unhealthy energy drinks to give them a boost. However, the negative effects of these drinks are well-documented and not worth the risk. We all desire increased energy, but it shouldn't come at the cost of our health.

Energy Drinks

Consuming an excessive amount of caffeinated energy drinks proves lethal to health consequences, especially for individuals with chronic heart conditions. A study has shown that over 4,500 poison control center calls were made by people who consumed too many of these hazardous drinks, and studies also indicate that energy drinks can significantly impact cardiac rhythm.

Daily consumption of energy drinks can lead to caffeine withdrawal-induced migraine headaches, as the body becomes dependent on the caffeine. Moreover, panic attacks, anxiety, and poor performance may result from consuming large quantities of energy drinks. Additionally, these drinks are intended to boost brain function but, ironically, can cause insomnia and other sleep issues. The high sugar content of energy drinks can exacerbate or even trigger type 2 Diabetes, and they can cause severe dehydration by depleting the body of essential fluids instead of replenishing them.

Finally, the high caffeine content of energy drinks can elevate blood pressure to dangerously high levels, putting individuals with high blood pressure at risk of strokes. Instead of resorting to toxic energy drinks and suffering the consequences, consider fruit juices as a healthy alternative that provides the body with the nutrients it requires to generate an abundance of energy.

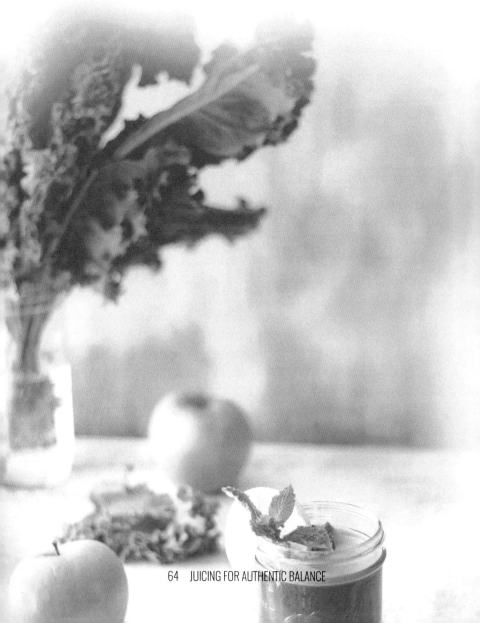

Chapter 8: Stop Suppressing Symptoms And Cleanse The Cells

Symptomology; let's start here. First, it is defined as "the set of symptoms characteristic of a particular medical condition or exhibited by a patient."

In my opinion, symptoms are indicators that something is amiss within the body, and they may resurface when the body is attempting to detoxify and heal itself. Regardless of whether we're actively detoxifying, symptoms will reappear if something isn't right.

What we consume directly affects our cells, which make up every part of the body—over 100 trillion of them, in fact. To truly heal from a condition, we must address it at the cellular level. That's why it's not wise to focus solely on symptoms. Instead, we must identify the root cause of the problem, which is damaging our cells. So, we must ask ourselves, "what is causing the damage?" This was my question as well, and let's take a step back and briefly examine this from a broader perspective.

When examining chemistry, there exist two types of solutions: alkaline and acid. It is the acidic solution that causes harm to the cells within the body. For the body to thrive, it is best to maintain an alkaline state.

The cells of the body are nourished by the blood, which gives them life. When we consume food, it is broken down by the microbiome within the duodenum, a small intestinal tract connected to the stomach. Absorption of phytonutrients occurs within this tract, and then the blood carries these nutrients to feed the cells.

Acid / Alkaline Food Comparison Chart

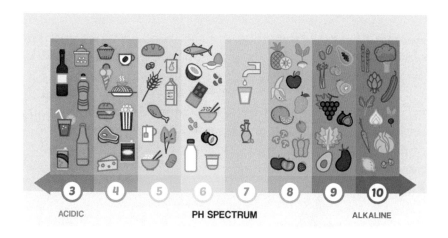

| 3 | 4 | 5 | 6 | 7 | 8 | 9 | 10 |

ACIDIC   PH SPECTRUM   ALKALINE

Health Benefits On Your Body

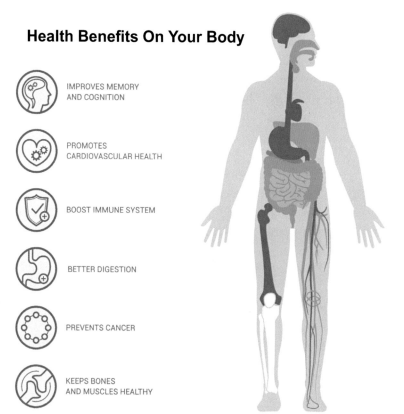

IMPROVES MEMORY AND COGNITION

PROMOTES CARDIOVASCULAR HEALTH

BOOST IMMUNE SYSTEM

BETTER DIGESTION

PREVENTS CANCER

KEEPS BONES AND MUSCLES HEALTHY

Acid / Alkaline Balanced Diet

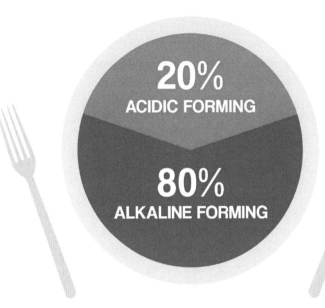

The 7 Most Alkaline Foods

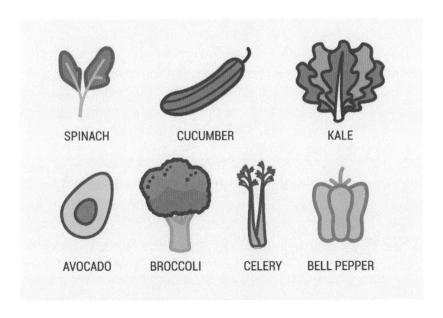

Although the body's blood is naturally alkaline, it requires acids to break down and digest food, absorb nutrients, and utilize them. If there are no acids present, the body will not function correctly, leading to difficulties in eliminating waste, often resulting in constipation for many Americans.

All the processes mentioned previously operate in an acidic environment. Let me elaborate further; to digest food, you need acids to break down proteins, and to absorb nutrients, you need acids to break down food for the microbiome to absorb them into the bloodstream. Moreover, acids break down nutrients, enabling the adrenal glands to utilize them. Therefore, without acids, it is impossible to break down food and eliminate metabolic cellular waste. Although the body functions in an acidic medium, maintaining the blood's alkaline balance is crucial.

It's important to note that a single symptom left untreated can negatively impact the entire body's function. That's why I repeatedly remind members of AB's community to ensure that their digestive, absorption, utilization, and elimination processes operate optimally. While I won't delve into the specifics of each process in this book, understand that they all work in conjunction with each other daily. Once you become a member, you'll hear me regularly discuss the four keys of the kingdom of our bodies and their functions during live sessions and other occasions. Eventually, understanding their purpose will become second nature.

It's important to understand that the acid side of the scale plays a vital role in bodily functions, just as the alkaline state does. Acids are necessary for the body to maintain balance, as they are produced through everyday activities such as eating. However, it's important to avoid consuming the wrong types of foods that contribute to the negative effects of acids. The key is to have more alkalinity in the body to achieve homeostasis.

To achieve this, you can refer to the charts provided within this book and strive to maintain an alkaline-based diet. It's important to note that most of the conditions we face are caused by the foods we eat. Therefore, we must avoid consuming certain foods, such as fried and processed foods, those high in salt and sugar, and those that are mucus-forming. These foods hinder the proper functioning of the body and contribute to the ailments people face. Remember, healing is simple, and a full alkaline diet can counteract the negative effects of acids in the body.

The reason behind this is that when harmful substances cannot be properly utilized by the body, they are expelled from the cells and end up accumulating in the joints. Over time, this build-up of toxins can cause damage to tendons, cartilages, and collagen—the main structural protein that forms the extracellular matrix of connective tissues in the body. Connective tissue refers to a group of tissues that provide internal support and maintain the shape of the body and its organs.

This includes various types of fibrous tissue, as well as recognizable variants such as bones, ligaments, tendons, and cartilage tissue. As a result of this damage, it becomes difficult for connective tissues to regenerate due to their lack of blood supply, minerals, and oxygen.

When there is an excess of acids between the joints, it leads to inflammation which can damage the connective tissues, resulting in pain and discomfort when moving. This is essentially what rheumatoid arthritis is—inflammation caused by the body's attempt to eliminate waste and mucus from consuming acidic foods.

To illustrate the importance of utilization, I have a personal example to share. I had a persistent issue with low iron levels, and all the supplements I took only made me feel worse. This caused a health crisis for me, as my body was unable to effectively eliminate toxins despite my efforts with various medications.

Only after I acquired my current knowledge did I realize that my adrenals required attention. The adrenals play a critical role in utilization, as they are responsible for transporting minerals to the blood and delivering them to various cells in the body. If you believe that you are anemic, as I did, it is more likely that your body is not utilizing nutrients properly due to adrenal fatigue. In our bodies, the imbalance caused by acids can lead to organ stress and inflammation, perpetuating an acidic state.

Achieving balance is crucial, and cellular regeneration involves eliminating toxins and promoting connective tissue regeneration. This can be achieved by consuming a lot of fluids, including fruit juices that contain H_3O_2, in addition to water. While water is still essential, the key to healing the body is to return to nature and stay hydrated by consuming fresh-pressed juices.

Furthermore, I emphasize the significance of incorporating juices that cleanse our lymphatic system, which functions like a filter for our body's waste disposal system, much like a filter in a fish tank. It's crucial to keep it clear to enable proper flow, as a blocked lymphatic system can hinder our body's ability to detoxify. It's crucial that you keep this at the forefront of your mind, as it's the key to maintaining proper flow of the four keys to our body.

Within AB's group, I also address several prevalent misconceptions related to nutrition and juicing, such as the idea that consuming high amounts of protein is advantageous, the notion that juices contain excessive amounts of sugar, and the belief that juicing is expensive. Additionally, I provide recommendations on how to combine ingredients for juicing and how to optimize your budget by avoiding the purchase of excess produce during the initial juicing stages. The group really goes into some intriguing topics, including the significance of including herbs within your daily juice regimen; explaining the comprehensive month-by-month herbal breakdown plan.

When you're prepared to implement my unique method, the steps will be presented more concisely when needed at each level. But even if you begin with the information presented in this book, it has the potential to alter the trajectory of your life. The journey has been simplified to avoid overwhelming you and to allow your body to adapt to the new lifestyle you'll be introducing.

At this stage, I think I've provided a clear enough foundation for you to see how crucial it is to change your eating habits. Food is the essence of life.

Eating healthy foods brings in specific frequencies as they are living entities, and this can make you think and live in an alkaline state. To live righteously, it is important to consume the suitable alkaline foods. We need to start behaving as we were genuinely and divinely created and treat ourselves accordingly. It's impossible to do so when we consume and function outside of balance. Operating and consuming food outside of a balanced state makes it impossible to treat ourselves as we were genuinely and divinely created. Instead, focus on providing your body with the right amount of fuel, including fruits, plants, vegetables, herbs, H_2O spring water, and H_3O_2 juice water, to initiate cellular regeneration.

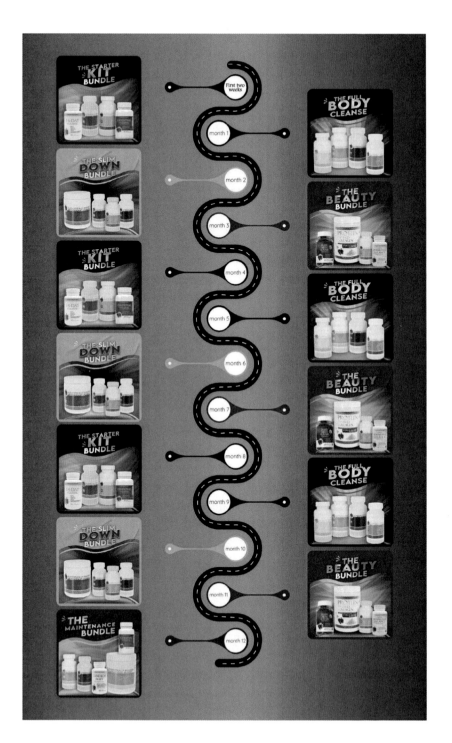

As previously mentioned, juicing is closely intertwined with every aspect of your being. This point is especially important as I emphasize it in this chapter. By following the Juicing For Authentic Balance System, you will notice a significant shift in focus from your physical state. Instead, you will be able to contemplate and pursue the things that bring you joy and excitement, including family, career, social life, and personal growth. As you embark on this journey, you will find yourself becoming more aligned with your purpose, and your daily life will become clearer and more fulfilling. You will be able to reflect on your existence, why you were created by a higher power, and the mission you are meant to fulfill. These deep reflections are difficult to achieve when your body is enslaved by unhealthy habits.

NEWS FLASH! Our bodies were not designed to be a prison. Instead, it should serve as an instrument for us to willingly express our divine nature during our time on earth. Regrettably, the things we consume have caused us to become enslaved to our bodies.

We have been violating the laws of nature, humanity, and the universe, resulting in a sowing and reaping process that is currently taking place. Let's take a moment to be honest with ourselves. All of the things we've been putting in our bodies, including negative thoughts and actions, are now having adverse effects.

Every action and decision, whether beneficial or not, carries consequences. These consequences can be positive or negative, regardless of how you view them. However, once you acknowledge and accept this fact, you can begin to recognize the current consequences of your actions and the reality they create. Realizing the significance of life and physical well-being can serve as a driving force to take charge of your mind, emotions, body, and energy. This moment marks true awakening and will encourage you to take the necessary steps to regain control and establish balance.

Viewing food as a source of information can heighten your awareness and consciousness of what you consume and how it affects your body. Food is a rich source of amino acids, trace minerals, and energy, which become incorporated into your body when consumed. Not to mention, eating clean or performing a juice fast can provide noticeable benefits such as a glowing complexion. This is due to the information and vitality contained in clean food and juice, which is nurtured by the sun and becomes an integral part of your being. Therefore, eating clean can be viewed as a way of charging your cellular structure and connecting with the Source.

During these times, it is crucial to recharge yourself daily. This will enable you to discover new opportunities in life and feel a natural energy flow when you surrender to the process. This energy is used to generate your cells. Personally, I experimented with eliminating certain foods during my healing journey, beginning with red meat and pork, then dairy. However, I continued to consume turkey, chicken, and fish, and I found it difficult to lose weight and experienced physical struggles. It wasn't until I completely cut out all animal products that my life began to improve significantly.

From my personal experience, I have found that cutting out meat and dairy products can be effective in regenerating cells and transforming one's life. In fact, I have not witnessed anyone achieve true cellular transformation while consuming animal products. If you genuinely want to transform and regenerate your cells, it is crucial to eliminate anything that obstructs the process. If you are uncertain about what to do, then stopping everything and reassessing is a clear sign that something is not working. Please note, however, that I am not suggesting that you must follow this lifestyle permanently. You can decide based on the positive changes you observe in your health. Instead of following many fad diets, I suggest "The Gaps Diet," which involve slowly eliminating and then reintroducing foods to identify problematic ones. I recommend prioritizing flooding and hydrating your body with H3O2 and adopting a lifestyle that includes clean foods, with an emphasis on fruits and vegetables.

Although I acknowledge that this chapter was lengthy, my intention was to emphasize these key ideas before transitioning to part three of the book. My hope is that you have gained a new perspective and feel enthusiastic about discovering how you can personally experience the beauty of the concepts discussed thus far. If that's the case, then it's time to introduce you to The Juicing for Authentic Balance System and explore my exclusive, innovative roadmap. So, what do you say? Are you prepared to take this next step?

" *Food is the essence of life.* "

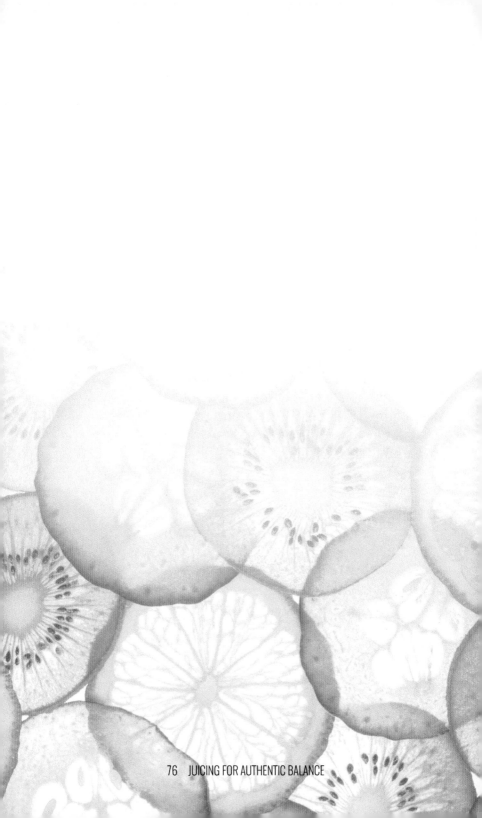

Part 3: All Roads Lead To Juicing For Authentic Balance

Chapter 9: Checkmate and A Quick History On How It All Began

Now that we have covered The State of the AB Community Address in Part 1 and The Power of Juicing in Part 2, it is time to examine the details of The Juicing for Authentic Balance in this final section. However, before we move forward, I want to reiterate these three words: Healing is Simple! You can rest assured that all the information you need will be presented in a clear and concise manner, making it easy to understand and implement immediately. If you are not ready to fully embrace juicing, that is perfectly acceptable. You may appreciate the concept, but perhaps you are not yet prepared for such a significant lifestyle change, or you may currently lack the necessary energy to incorporate it into your daily routine.

It's great that you're honest with yourself and making decisions that work best for you. However, I want to highlight that this could be the perfect time to start incorporating juice into your diet. Consuming your regular food may result in the accumulation of toxins, leading to a decline in energy levels and overall wellbeing. Providing your body with the necessary nutrients through juicing can help counteract these effects. Even if you're not ready to make a complete lifestyle change, adding at least one glass of fresh-pressed juice to your routine can make a significant difference.

Perhaps you're hesitant to start juicing because you feel like it's too complicated and you don't have enough time in your day to add something else to your routine. That's understandable, and it's perfectly okay to start slowly. As the great Chinese philosopher Lao Tzu once said, "A journey of a thousand miles begins with a single step." By embarking on this journey with me and those within the AB community, you'll see just how easy it is to implement this system and start living *The AB Way*.

I'll guide you through each step of the journey and simplify the road ahead, starting with the simple act of having one juice for breakfast and eating well for the rest of the day. Sounds doable, right?

Before I dive into the details of how the Juicing for Authentic Balance system operates, let me share the story of how I came to develop this strategy. By understanding the context behind this proprietary system, you will gain valuable insights into how AB's methodology can be effective for you as well.

You see, let me inform you that Juicing for Authentic Balance wasn't my first attempt. Prior to this, I had created a program called The AB Life Program, where I made mistakes and learned lessons that led me to develop my current juicing strategy.

In the previous program, I aimed to restore various aspects of participants' lives, including health, self-esteem, stress management, and more. However, the program suffered from information overload and provided too many options, including different nutritional tiers for meat eaters, vegetarians, vegans, and plant-based diets.

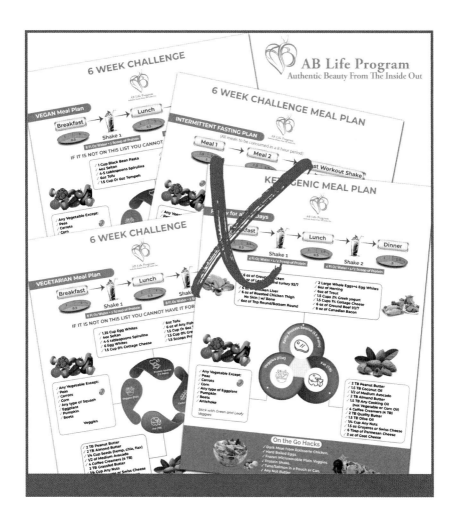

However, when I discovered that I had parasites and learned which foods were actually feeding them, I realized that I could no longer continue with my usual habits. It didn't seem right to endorse strategies that were not serving my body, especially since many women in my community were facing similar issues. As a result, I had to step back and take a break from it all due to my health issues and lack of energy. Later, when I returned, I made a video for the group and explained the situation. I gave everyone the option to join me on my new journey, which was inspired by divine intervention, which became my juicing evolution.

To sum it up, I wanted to share my realizations with others, but encountered another setback after overcoming the *Candida* issue. Despite my efforts to address the problem, I experienced persistent symptoms such as mood swings, uncontrollable cravings, and difficulty losing weight.

As my health declined, I sought help from an endocrinologist and was diagnosed with thyroid and adrenal issues. It was a miserable experience. As I mentioned earlier in this book, I didn't feel like myself and sought the assistance of my colon hydrotherapist, who discovered that I had parasites during our session. It felt like my world had come to a halt.

After discovering that my body was infested with parasites, I embarked on a rigorous mission to eradicate them by researching scientific studies and literature on parasites and their behavior. My lack of connection with my body over the years had taken a toll on me, and I knew I had to take practical steps to restore my health. I eliminated all animal products and foods that fed mucus and yeast, and underwent a thorough cleansing process.

During this time, I stumbled upon information about the detoxifying properties of certain fruits, and an ad for a Juicing Certification program caught my attention. Although my initial intention was to gain more knowledge to aid in my healing journey, I found myself fully immersed in the program and began juicing right away. The amount of information I learned was astounding, and I completed the program and received my accreditation in record time. This was the turning point in my life where my true transformation began.

I spent a year and a half in isolation, undergoing various fruit cleanses and exploring the depths of each healing session. Things initially worsened before they improved, but each time I did a juice cleanse, I felt like I was making progress. The excess weight vanished, my skin cleared up, and symptoms like irritability, brain fog, lack of energy, fatigue, and lack of clarity began to fade away. I continued to get colonics to aid in the cleansing and healing process. After over a year and a half on this journey, I was thrilled to be told during one of my appointments that no parasites were detected. This was the day I had been waiting for.

Because of the profound impact juicing has had on my life after years of suffering, I used the knowledge I gained as a Certified Juice Therapist to spread this message to as many people as possible who are seeking change on a deep, cellular level. I comprehend the power of juicing, and my life is a reflection of it.

That's my story. Now, let's explore the three levels of AB's transitional strategy.

> *" A journey of a thousand miles begins with a single step. "*

Chapter 10: The Three Levels Of Juicing
For *Authentic Balance*

To begin, I will explain the three levels that drive our methodology. In the upcoming chapters, I will explore AB's model extensively and illustrate how you can integrate it into your life. Prior to examining the upcoming chart, let me give a brief summary of how simple this transitional system is. During level 1, swap your typical breakfast with a juice, and if you don't have a juicer yet, have a smoothie or a bowl of fruit instead. For lunch, opt for a vegetable-rich meal such as salads, vegetable stir-fry, fresh veggies, or vegetable soup. Dinner is your choice, but be mindful of portion control. Eliminate fried, packaged, and processed foods, and replace snacks with fruit, juice, or smoothies.

During level 2, have juice for breakfast and another juice with lunch instead of a veggie-heavy meal. For dinner, avoid all animal products. You can still consume fruits throughout the day and have more juice or smoothies if needed.

Moving onto level 3, you will embark on an all-juice cleanse journey. You should aim to cleanse four times a year, and the AB's 28-day Transitional Process should take place every quarter. If this is your first time and you are not experiencing any significant health issues, begin with a 5-day cleanse, then progress to a 7-day cleanse, next time around, a 10-day cleanse, and conclude your final cleanse of the year with a 14-day cleanse.

If you face challenging health problems, you should have a customized plan that takes into account all prescribed medications, which should be approved by your practicing medical physician. Further information on this will be available in the Facebook group.

Let's Navigate Through The Different Levels

Level (days 1–7) 1st Week Moderate Transition

- **UPON WAKING** – 4oz fresh pressed lemon shot or mixed with equal portion of distilled or spring water.
- **BREAKFAST** – pick any of the following: 1. fruits consisting of the three different categories; 2. smoothie of your choice; 3. fresh pressed juice
- **MID MORNING** – fruits from either of the three categories
- **LUNCH** – pick any of the following: 1. alkaline salad made with watercress, arugula, romaine, kale, dandelion greens, green leaf lettuce (toppings: cucumbers, tomatoes, olives, avocado, alfalfa, sprouts, onions, peppers, any vinaigrette with or without lemon, NO cream-based dressings); 2. vegan bowl of choice, any type of vegetables (raw or sauteed stir-fry), or vegetable soup; 3. green smoothie or juice
- **MID AFTERNOON** – fruits from either of the three categories
- **DINNER**– your choice

Level (days 8–14) 2nd Week Advanced Transition

- **UPON WAKING** – 4oz fresh pressed lemon shot or mixed with equal portion of distilled or spring water.
- **BREAKFAST** – pick any of the following: 1. fruits consisting of the three different categories; 2. smoothie of your choice; 3. fresh pressed juice
- **MID MORNING** – fruits from either of the three categories (30 mins before lunch: 4oz fresh pressed lemon shot or mixed with equal portion of distilled or spring water.)
- **LUNCH** – pick any of the following: 1. fruits consisting of the three different categories; 2. smoothie of your choice; 3. fresh pressed juice
- **MID AFTERNOON** – fruits from either of the three categories
- **DINNER**– your choice (but NO animal products or any byproduct from such)

Level ③ Weeks 3 and 4 Intense Transition

- **UPON WAKING** – 4oz fresh pressed lemon shot or mixed with equal portion of distilled or spring water.
- **8AM**– green tea
- **10AM** – 32oz of juice
- **11AM** – 24–32oz of distilled or spring water
- **1PM** – 32oz of juice
- **2PM** – 24–32oz of distilled or spring water
- **3PM** – 32oz of juice
- **5PM** – 24–32oz of distilled or spring water
- **7–8PM** – cup of herbal detox tea or herbal detox supplement

Level 1: 1st Week Moderate Transition

The reason for the lack of inspiration and results in your previous health journey is often due to overcomplicating things. The solution is simple: follow a system, stay on track, and avoid getting bogged down in too many processes. My previous approach had too many moving parts, which can cause one to become uninspired and struggle to achieve results.

To combat this, I've created a new way of thinking about cleansing and healing our bodies that makes it easier to implement. It may not happen overnight, but the starting process is not overwhelming. It involves knowing what to eliminate from your diet and what to consume more of. In the following sections, I will guide you through my entire transitional strategy step-by-step.

Transitioning

The primary goal at level 1 is to acclimate yourself to juicing and consume more fruits. The second goal is to shift your mindset towards food and become more conscious of what you put in your body. For some individuals, jumping straight into an all-juice cleanse may not be feasible or they may require guidance for alternative options.

This could be due to intense cravings, digestive disorders, exhaustion, blood sugar difficulties, or serious lymphatic issues that necessitate a more gradual cleanse. In such cases, I recommend starting at level 1 before moving on to an all-juice detox, especially if you are transitioning from the Standard American Diet (SAD).

The duration of time spent at level 1 varies depending on the individual, and I suggest alternating between level 1 and 2 as needed before progressing to level 3. More information on this is provided during our live gatherings or in the Facebook group.

There are two main goals to keep in mind. Firstly, it's important to observe how your body responds to the changes you're making. Secondly, when you gradually start incorporating solid foods back into your diet after consuming more juices, it's crucial to be mindful of what you're eating and avoid reverting to old habits. Once you've progressed to level 2 and have adopted a cleaner eating pattern, it's essential to maintain this habit. While some individuals may not experience any issues when reintroducing solid foods, others may encounter digestive discomfort. It's essential to be aware of your body's reactions and trust your intuition.

Level 2: 2nd Week Advanced Transition

Once you reach the second week, you will have had the opportunity to start juicing and become more familiar with the process. While you may not have fully mastered it, you should have a basic understanding. Level 2 involves consuming more juice in order to amplify the results achieved in level 1.

During level 2, you will have juices for breakfast and lunch while also incorporating clean eating. For dinner, animal products are eliminated, and the focus is on a high plant-based meal. Simplifying dinner and eating clean is also an option during level 1 before transitioning to level 2. As you approach level 3, it's important to be firm with yourself and avoid having withdrawals.

This approach is highly strategic, and it's crucial to be mindful of what you consume at this stage. There is a science behind it all, which will be discussed in chapter 11.

Level 3: Weeks 3 and 4 Intense Transition

On level 3, the focus is solely on an ALL-juice cleanse, which is the starting point for going deeper into your body and repairing yourself from within. If you feel the need to eat something at the beginning of this level, I highly recommend only consuming highly astringent fruits like melons and citrus fruits listed on the fruit chart in the next chapter. However, the ultimate goal is to work towards consuming all juices. This phase is like a Juice Feast Party!

Levels 1 and 2 were simply preparation by eliminating certain foods, incorporating juices into your current lifestyle, and getting you physically and mentally ready for what's to come in this level.

In the past few years, I have extensively studied this methodology, specifically focusing on the juices that are ideal to begin with and gradually increasing their potency to extract mucus and acid from the cells. In the upcoming chapter, I will explain in detail why it is necessary to eliminate certain foods during this process, the significance of consuming the right ingredients, and why it is crucial to prioritize specific produce for juicing.

Oh, and by the way! After completing the all-juice cleanse cycle, level 2 is recommended as a reference point to achieve continuous *Authentic Balance* between your quarterly cleanses. Let's proceed.

Chapter 11: Purpose Of The Transitional Process

Let's start talking about the purpose of this process, and how my methodology can practically benefit you. As you continue reading, I will help you gain a better understanding of a few things before embarking on your own juicing journey.

Before we proceed, I would like to express my gratitude for allowing me to be a part of your journey. I have put in a lot of effort into this proprietary method to provide tools and resources to prevent others from going through what I have been through. My goal is to help you and others on your journey of cleansing and healing.

I firmly believe that proper nutrition is key to achieving healing. AB's Transitional Program aims to change your internal environment from an acidic one, which can cause unwanted outcomes, to an alkaline environment. This process removes the obstructions that cause symptoms leading to many "dis-eases." The goal is to give your glands, cells, tissues, organs, and systems the chance to regenerate and function optimally.

Let's take a step back from what you've been taught for a moment. While I appreciate the intentions of doctors and health professionals, I want to emphasize that healing is absolutely possible. I've personally experienced the power of detoxification, as have members of my community and clients.

What you eat and what you eliminate from your diet both play important roles in your body's ability to heal. As a holistic practitioner, my aim is to guide people towards finding *Authentic Balance* through cleansing from within. Whether your goal is to address a specific ailment, make a lifestyle change, or rid your body of accumulated toxins, the ultimate goal remains the same: CLEANSE TO HEAL. I've said it before and I'll say it again, CLEANSE TO HEAL, CLEANSE TO HEAL, CLEANSE TO HEAL. Are we clear? Great!

Base Rules

To facilitate the detoxification process and promote healing, it is crucial to make dietary adjustments. It's important to avoid consuming items that can hinder the process, such as animal products (including dairy), fried and processed foods, packaged goods, wheat, gluten, regular pasta, crackers, white bread, white rice, snack chips, corn, breakfast cereals, potatoes, soy, processed and sugary drinks.

Remember: I can't express this enough; detoxifying your body requires getting rid of acidic, dehydrating, mucus-forming, and lymphatic-blocking substances. These toxins can cause glands, organs, and tissues to fail. In order to create an alkaline environment for regeneration, you need to consume only highly hydrating and astringent foods to eliminate toxins in your body.

As you follow AB's process, you will gradually eliminate animal products and increase your intake of raw foods and juices. The primary objective is to eliminate specific foods that cause mucus-forming activities in an acidic body. To achieve an alkaline state, focus on consuming alkaline foods. You deserve a life of energy and vitality! If you're here, it's because you've held on to a lifestyle that has caused pain for too long. Now is the time to heal and detoxify your body for cell regeneration, making everything, including healing, possible!

Purpose

The body possesses incredible healing capabilities once it receives the necessary attention and resources to undergo a detoxifying process. Juice fasting, for instance, allows the body to take a break from the digestion of solid foods and focus on self-healing. The benefits of cleansing extend beyond physical health and into the realm of mental and spiritual well-being. It's important to note that during a juice feast, you will still consume enough calories and nutrition.

By ingesting juices, the nutrients are rapidly absorbed into the bloodstream, freeing up the body's energy reserves, which would otherwise be expended on digesting food. Juicing is an effective method for cleansing the body of mucus, mucoid plaque, and undigested toxins, which are the sources of all sicknesses.

In addition, high fruit consumption and juice feasting can transform one's outlook on life, leading to an appreciation of the body and a better understanding of how previous lifestyle choices may have been detrimental. It is the single most important action you can take for your health and well-being. Let's get it!

Healing "Dis" Eases

In order to heal any illness, it is important to prioritize the three main causes of sickness: excessive acidity, blockages, and weakness in organs and glands. These factors are often at the root of people's illnesses. When working towards healing the body and addressing these underlying causes of disease, a clean diet is the most critical aspect to focus on. This is because a clean diet creates a well-hydrated environment that can help remove mucus, parasites, acids, toxins, and chemicals from the body. Additionally, a clean diet can provide the necessary alkalinity that the body needs to repair damaged tissue in all organs and glands.

The raw detoxifying diet utilizes the healing properties of fruit, with the goal of gradually transitioning individuals to a consumption pattern that is primarily fruit-based and tailored to their preferences. Fruit is known to be the most effective food for drawing out mucus, stimulating the lymphatic system, energizing cells, and repairing the nervous system and glands. Additionally, consuming fruit requires the least amount of digestive energy, which can be redirected to repairing the body. To successfully cure any illness, an all-raw diet is crucial. For those who are unsure of how to start, a progressive level chart can be followed, beginning with a diet that is 50% raw, including fresh-pressed juice.

Level 1 and level 2 of the raw detoxifying diet involve consuming juices for breakfast and lunch, while level 3 (Eating All Raw) only requires drinking fresh pressed juice and eating fruits. Please refer to the 3-level chart for more details.

Note: Remember that "raw" and/or "clean eating" refers to any whole fruit or vegetable that hasn't been cooked or processed. More on this discussed within the group.

When it comes to your raw diet, you have the flexibility to make it as simple or complex as you want. However, keep in mind that the simpler your diet is, the faster your recovery will be. I have worked with clients who have found it challenging to transition to juicing right away, and they required transitional stages. That is why I have developed this process strategically, so it can assist people at all stages of their cleansing process.

Transitional Process

The consumption of meat, dairy products, and eggs can be detrimental to human health, even though they are commonly used in recipes that are perceived as healthy. Many people are not aware that these foods may be the root cause of their health issues. Eliminating them from your diet can lead to noticeable improvements in your body's healing and restoration.

Plant-based substitutes can aid in your cleansing goals but I strongly recommend clean eating for healing and rejuvenation. It is important to be cautious with substitutions for meat and dairy products and avoid overuse. Although they can be beneficial for moving away from animal products, they are not particularly beneficial for cleansing purposes. During this process, it is crucial to proceed with care and avoid overdoing it since the most harmful products have already been removed.

Why High Fruits?

The regenerative properties of fruits can positively impact the neurological system, and their astringent nature makes them the most powerful food for removing impurities from the body. Harmful substances that are acidic, toxic, or congested can obstruct the body and lead to cell, tissue, organ, and gland degeneration. Fruits can help eliminate cellular waste, mucus, chemicals, mucoid plaque, neurotoxins, colon debris, parasites, fungi, heavy metals, and drug residues.

It is interesting to note that human anatomy is more suited towards a frugivorous diet in comparison to other diets found in nature. Our digestive system, vision, ability to identify ripe fruit, and dexterous fingers all support this idea. By focusing on a fruit-based diet, you can experience transformative changes in your physical, mental, emotional, and spiritual well-being. As you continue on this journey, you will uncover more insights about this subject.

Fruit Chart

Astringents: DETOXIFY AND PULL ACID FROM THE CELLS:
apples, grapefruit, grapes, key limes, lemons, mangoes, oranges, peaches, pears, pineapples, pomegranates, tangerines

Antioxidants: OXYGENATE AND PROTECT THE CELLS:
cherries, bearberries, blackberries, blueberries, elderberries, goji berries, juniper berries, mulberries, persimmons, raspberries, rosehip berries, strawberries

Phyto-nutrients: REBUILD AND ENERGIZE THE CELLS:
bitter melon, cantaloupe, cucumber, honey globe melon, honeydew melon, horned melon, musk melon, papaya, watermelon, winter melon

Please refer back to the fruit chart, as I would like to explain the significance of consuming highly astringent and detoxifying fruits during your detoxification process.

Astringent fruits are the most effective foods to consume during detoxification, as they work to eliminate toxins, mucus, acids, parasites, pathogens, yeast, and fungus from the body on an intracellular level. These fruits flood the lymphatic system and are considered extremely powerful in detoxifying the body. After being filtered by the liver and kidney, they release toxins through urination, bowel movements, and the skin. Fruits are excellent sources of electrical phytonutrients and easily digestible foods, consisting mainly of monosaccharides that provide the energy necessary for cellular functions. It is no wonder why I feel so energized lately!

Now, let's focus on detoxification. The detoxification process involves the elimination of acids in the cells, which can be aided by consuming grapes, particularly dark ones with seeds that are organic. Grapes have a potent astringency property that is beneficial in detoxifying the lymphatic system. Alternatively, lemon and/or key limes are great astringents that can benefit the lymphatic system and eliminate acids at the cellular level.

The berry family is rich in antioxidants, including blueberries, blackberries, raspberries, strawberries, and mulberries. These fruits are oxygenators, providing energy and oxygen to your body's cells while also safeguarding them. Don't overlook the juniper berry, which is excellent for eliminating toxins from the kidneys and promoting their proper functioning. Elderberry is also highly beneficial for cleansing the lymphatic system and removing mucus.

Moving on to melons, they are packed with phytonutrients and are ideal for rebuilding the body's cellular structure while following an all-fruit diet. Watermelon, cantaloupe, and honeydew are detoxifiers that are also great for hydrating your body, which can aid absorption once your lymphatic system has been cleansed and your malabsorption issues have been resolved. It's crucial to remember that digestion, absorption, utilization for assimilation, and elimination are all important steps in the healing process of our bodies.

If you're looking to cleanse your pancreas and manage insulin levels due to diabetes, bitter melon is worth a try. It has an extremely bitter taste that you won't soon forget. It's essential to have a sufficient supply of raw fruits, vegetables, and greens available.
The saying "if you fail to plan, you plan to fail" is particularly

relevant here because cleansing begins with proper nutrition, and preparation is key to healing. The fruit chart's fruits should be available at all times to hydrate your body and help eliminate toxins.

It's crucial to remember that without an alkaline and hydrated environment, no tissues, organs, or glands can repair themselves. The fruit chart's fruits can help you achieve the optimal hydrating and alkaline environment necessary for regeneration to occur.

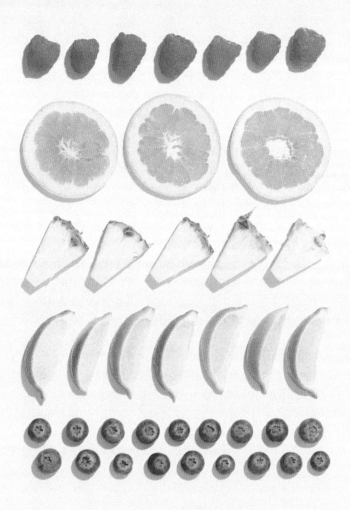

Chapter 12: Preparing For Your Juicing Journey

Getting Geared Up for Your Fast

To start, it is essential to have a juicer that is not only enjoyable and easy to operate but also easy to clean. I highly recommend a Slow Press Cold Juicer over a Centrifugal one, as it preserves the nutrients by not heating them up and is the most high-quality and low-maintenance juicer available.

You can find AB's Juicer at **www.abjuicer.com**.

Make it a priority to obtain a colon cleanser as soon as possible. Remember that anything you don't eliminate accumulates. If you're experiencing difficulties in this area, focus on having regular bowel movements at least three times a day by using a colon cleanser and consuming clean foods.

If you haven't already, be sure to get AB's Herbal Starter Kit Bundle. Once you start eliminating correctly (which those pills will help you with), you'll enter the detox phase. Proper elimination is vital during cleansing, and it may make you feel terrible at times. Learn to take breaks and relax. Rest is crucial during this time, so don't feel guilty about it. You're not being lazy; you're healing. Give yourself some credit and allow yourself to relax.

Recommended Daily Juices

During your juice fast, both your intuition and human instinct will become stronger, allowing you to determine how much your body needs simply by listening to it. On levels 1 and 2, aim to work up to consuming at least two 32-oz mason jars of juice.

About Water

Although water is not strictly necessary during a juice fast, you may sometimes feel a natural craving for it. If you do choose to drink water, it's best to opt for spring or distilled varieties. Keep in mind that consuming water while on a juice fast can lead to feelings of fullness before you've consumed enough calories, which can trigger hunger pangs.

During this time, it's important to rely on juices made from raw fruits and vegetables to provide you with the nourishment you need. Additionally, you can incorporate unpasteurized coconut water or homemade nut "milk" into your routine, especially when you reach level 3 of the fast.

While nut milk can be a soothing way to end your day, it's best not to overdo it, as the fat content can impede the detoxification process. Ultimately, it is essential to closely observe and heed the signals your body gives, and modify your approach accordingly.

Levels Of Detox

As you embark on this transformative journey, you will experience a rapid healing process that involves the release of both physical toxins and emotional baggage. Be prepared for ups and downs, as the detoxification process can be an emotional rollercoaster. It's best to avoid making too many plans in advance, as you never know how you'll feel. This is why I isolated myself for over a year—to take my healing seriously. While we'll always be on a path of healing, following the plan precisely will bring you to a place of greater self-awareness and understanding. Prepare yourself and embrace the process.

Levels Of Detox Chart

Level 1	WATER FASTING	ACCELERATES DETOX
Level 2	MONO FRUIT JUICE	
Level 3	FRUIT JUICE	
Level 4	FRUIT SMOOTHIES	
Level 5	100% FRUITS, BERRIES, MELONS	
Level 6	(BREAKFAST) FRUITS, BERRIES, MELONS (LUNCH/DINNER) LARGE SALAD	
Level 7	GREEN SMOOTHIES OR JUICES	SLOWS DETOX
Level 8	RAW FRUITS AND VEGETABLES	

We've been using food and pharmaceuticals to numb our emotions and have become experts at managing symptoms, as discussed in earlier chapters. It's time to get to know ourselves and address the underlying issues causing our symptoms. Cleansing can bring up uncomfortable feelings that we've been masking with food and medications. It's time to face them head-on so we can live our lives to the fullest and truly heal.

When you enter a healing crisis, also known as die-off symptoms, you may experience various discomforts such as nausea, brain fog, and scattered thoughts. Although it's unpleasant, these symptoms are an indication that your body is getting rid of toxins, and it's a part of the healing process. To remind yourself of this, you can repeat it to yourself whenever you encounter such symptoms.

If you're not experiencing any symptoms, it means you need to increase your fruit or juice intake. As you go through several healing crises, you'll begin to realize that you're healing. Symptoms can last up to 72 hours, during which you can ease up a bit on your juice intake and switch to green juices or smoothies to detoxify at a comfortable rate. Throughout your journey, I will explain various strategies to speed up or slow down your detoxification process, which can take years. However, a proactive juice feast can heal many discomforts and diseases in as little as a month or so. It's important to trust the process, but it's not for the faint of heart.

Get Those Bowels Moving

Throughout your juice fast, it is essential to have regular bowel movements, ideally between 2 to 4 times per day. To help with this, you may consider using a colon cleanse supplement, detox tea, or psyllium. If you are not eliminating waste frequently, gradually increase your intake of psyllium husk to three times per day over three days, taking one tablespoon each time.

Additionally, you can increase the frequency of drinking laxative tea to twice per day, using two packets per tea (depending on the brand). For more information on these supplements, please refer to the sections on the following page.

Detox Assistance

In our Facebook group, we provide a detailed list of essential items that can aid in managing the uncomfortable detox symptoms that often arise during cleansing. You don't have to endure the same struggle that I did. I am here to support you in every way possible and help you avoid feeling unwell and down. There are products available that can aid in the absorption of toxins that are attempting to exit your body, so rest assured, I have got you covered.

Where To Shop

It's recommended to source your produce locally if possible, such as through farmer's markets or personal connections with growers. The benefits of freshly picked fruit from a tree cannot be overstated, especially for the neurological and endocrine systems. If local farmer's markets are not available in your area, seek out the highest-quality fruits, greens, and veggies you can find. Many natural and organic grocers, supermarkets, and health food stores offer a variety of produce, much of which is organic and pesticide-free. For the freshest and finest quality, look for produce that is organic, local, tree-ripened, and picked on the same day.

While organic, locally grown, tree-ripened, and same-day-picked produce will offer the freshest and best quality, it's still possible to cleanse and heal your body without access to these options. I have worked with individuals who had limited access to organic options and still experienced successful detoxification and healing. Fruits are particularly powerful in this regard, and even those with limited access to organic options can still benefit from frozen or dried fruits, as well as common fruits like apples, oranges, bananas, and local varieties. The key is to find what works for you and to stay committed to your healing process.

Buying Organic

It is advisable to prioritize purchasing organic produce, as fruits and vegetables sprayed with pesticides can be detrimental to the body, particularly for those with compromised nervous systems. If buying organic is not feasible for all items, consider purchasing organic thin-skinned fruits and vegetables such as grapes, berries, apples, and greens. Thick-skinned fruits like oranges, melons, and avocados, however, do not necessarily have to be organic as pesticides tend to accumulate in the peeled skin.

The "Dirty Dozen vs The Clean 15"

In my humbled opinion, the list of fruits and vegetables falling under the "Dirty Dozen" and "The Clean 15" categories exceeds 12 and 15, respectively. However, the decision to buy conventionally or organically ultimately rests with you. Additionally, you can purchase a fruit and vegetable wash that is free of pesticides.

The "Dirty Dozen" category includes nectarines, imported snap beans, potatoes, strawberries, spinach, kale, collard and mustard greens, apples, grapes, berries, bell peppers, peaches, cherries, celery, pears, and tomatoes. These are the products that are more likely to be exposed to toxins such as pesticides.

On the other hand, the "Clean 15" category includes pineapple, onion, cabbage, avocado, frozen sweet peas, sweet corn, papaya, mango, eggplant, melons, kiwi, grapefruit, and sweet potatoes. These products are typically considered safe to purchase conventionally as they have a shell or a hard outer covering.

Kitchen Gadgets

Having the right kitchen utensils can greatly simplify your experience in the kitchen, particularly if you are following a raw vegan diet. By using the appropriate tools, you can save time, become more creative with recipes, and even enhance your detoxification process by making easier-to-digest juices and smoothies. I find these tools to be particularly beneficial, and I suggest expanding your kitchen tool collection as soon as possible.

Juicer

One of the essential tools for a raw vegan diet is a juicer. The AB juicer is an excellent choice because it is versatile and perfect for beginners. Despite its small size, it has a powerful motor that can extract a substantial amount of juice from fruits and vegetables while leaving behind dry pulp. Although it is a slow-press juicer, it produces high-quality juice, including grape, green, and watermelon juice, which are great for cleansing. Additionally, it can handle a variety of other juicing tasks. If you prefer a faster juicing method, you may want to consider centrifugal juicers.

Mason Jars

Using mason jars is an excellent way to preserve the freshness of juices and smoothies. While the metal covers that often come with them can corrode, there are many different lids available that can be easily swapped out. These jars come in a variety of sizes to meet your storage needs, whether you want to store a large amount of juice for several days, pour your drink into a jar, or keep your salad dressing for the following day. They are an essential tool to have on your detox journey.

Insulated Travel Container

To ensure success during your journey, it's crucial to prepare accordingly. A travel container with a capacity of at least 32 ounces is a must-have, although smaller or larger sizes are also available depending on your needs.

Sharp Knives

Having sharp kitchen knives is also essential, as they can significantly reduce the time required to prepare produce for juicing.

Lemon Squeezer

For those times when you need a quick squeeze of citrus in your juices, a lemon squeezer is incredibly useful. It can extract the most juice from your lemons and limes without having to juice multiple fruits for maximum detoxification power.

Strainer

A strainer is also an important tool to have on hand, particularly when you are on level 3 of juice feasting when you want to give your digestive system a break. Placing the strainer on top of your container before consuming your juice allows you to remove any additional pulp.

Preparation Is Key

To adhere to the detoxifying protocol, it's critical to plan ahead by ensuring you have enough fruits stocked in your kitchen for at least three days. Personally, I prefer to purchase fresh produce twice a week. Additionally, it's important to eliminate any tempting foods from your household during the detoxification process, as you may experience moments of weakness and intense cravings that could derail your progress. It's better to avoid processed foods or other tempting cheats altogether to help you resist these cravings.

Staying Committed

Strive for a sense of well-being, which will lead to complete restoration of your body. Your health should be your top priority, and only you can take control of how you feel in your own body. You have the power to cleanse and heal yourself. By making daily choices towards health, you can create health and vitality. Just as many of us have contributed to our current poor health through bad dietary choices and lifestyle practices, we can also turn it around.

Your current state of being is largely influenced by several factors including your nutrition, lifestyle choices, environment, social connections, daily thoughts and emotions, and overall level of enjoyment. These factors all impact your physical body. While changing your food choices is an important part of cleansing, it's only one piece of the puzzle. Other aspects of your life should not be ignored. This is why I tell people, "My only job is to truly awaken you so that you can return to your true self," and that applies to every area of your life. Following the advice in this book is a great starting point!

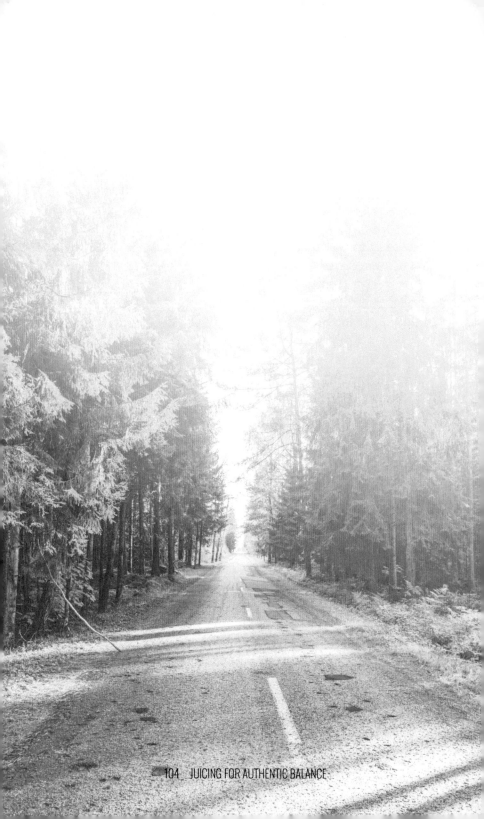

Now What?

Well, we have come to the end of this road together, and I truly hope that you have gained numerous benefits from this book.

Now, the next step is simple: keep moving forward.

You can choose to seek assistance or pursue it independently, but keep pushing ahead.

While the Juicing For Authentic Balance System may not immediately resolve all of your current problems, it's a great starting point that can provide you with the longevity and various other benefits that you are seeking.

If you decide you desire help, please contact us at **www.juicewithmisty.com** and let's discuss your situation. I strongly believe in what we do, and I am proud to say so.

I acknowledge that you possess something valuable to contribute to the world, and I would feel privileged to assist you in bringing everything together, beginning with your *Authentic Body*, where health and wellness emanate from within you. I would be delighted to accompany you on your journey, supporting you to implement all the knowledge you have gained from this book while also holding you responsible and providing encouragement along the way. If you're interested in exploring further, let's discuss how we can work together!

Here's to your tremendous success!

Forever and Always Authentically Yours,

Misty Angelique

About the Author

Misty Angelique, also known as "The Authentic Juice Queen," is on a mission to help many discover and embrace their true authenticity.

Juicing has been instrumental in my personal journey, not only for cleansing my body of physical ailments but also for achieving success in areas of life that had held me back for too long. My aim is to demonstrate what authenticity looks like in every aspect of life, as I strongly believe that "Authenticity is Legacy."

Aside from my various titles, I relish experiencing an *Authentic Balance* lifestyle. However, this wasn't always the case. After being forced to retire due to my medical conditions, I created Authentically Branded Hair & Skin Care over a decade ago, which eventually led to the formation of my company, Authentically Branded Solutions.

Despite my efforts, my medical conditions only worsened, and I was misdiagnosed with an autoimmune disorder, leading to numerous hospitalizations, medications, and a "mystery case" label. Seeking natural remedies and holistic approaches, I discovered that my body was overrun by yeast overgrowth and parasites. Despite trying various diet plans, nothing seemed to work.

Determined to find a solution, I pursued a Juicing Certification Program and realized the wonders of juicing for cleansing and restoring the body to an alkaline state. After experiencing the transformative power of juicing, I set out to help as many people as possible struggling with physical ailments or seeking a healthier lifestyle.

Not only has juicing helped me restore my health, shed unwanted pounds, reduce inflammation, clear acne, improve digestion, and alleviate various health concerns, but it can also help you achieve *Authentic Balance*, or #theABway. I am fully dedicated to supporting and guiding you on your wellness journey, with a focus on...

...authentically awakening your true self every step of the way.

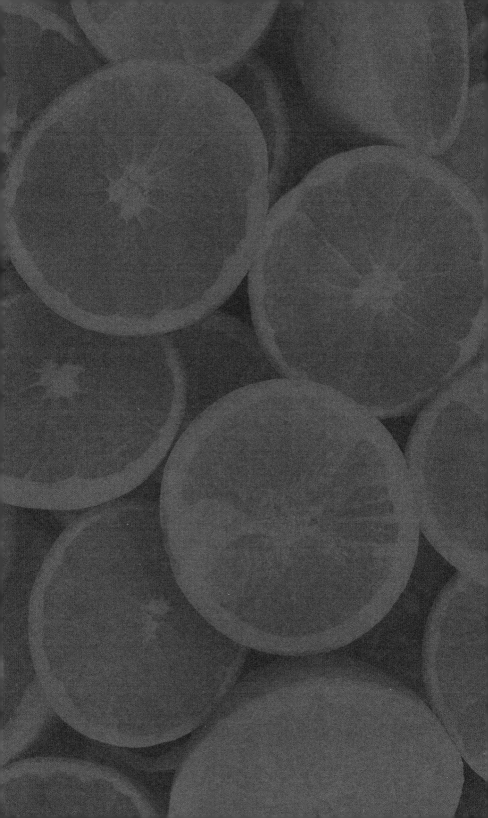

Made in United States
Orlando, FL
04 October 2024

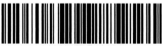

52365971R00064